Introduction

We live in a time of significant challenges and opportunities across all parts of society, including healthcare. As we navigate uncertain times and potential crises, we call on all individuals, communities, and nations to unite around shared values. The first of these values is that healthcare is a fundamental human right. We must work together to create a healthcare system that is sustainable, equitable, and innovative. This book is designed to serve as both a manifesto and a manual, fulfilling two essential functions: defining the Elevate Health Community and providing a step-by-step guide to enable anyone to create a health market for their community.

Defining the Elevate Health Community

We envision a global community of stakeholders—patients, caregivers, builders, public health officials, and citizens—collaborating to create the healthcare system of the future. This community operates like other successful open-source projects: united around shared values but diverse in implementation strategies. Anyone can join, contribute, and benefit, regardless of their geographic location, political affiliation, religion, or cultural background.

The Step-by-Step Manual

The middle five chapters of the book constitute a comprehensive implementation guide for building an Elevate Health market to benefit any community. This manual outlines the key steps to take when bootstrapping a new health market for a community, be it large or small. In Chapter 4, we explain the importance of establishing shared values and foundational beliefs for the community. These values and beliefs serve as the guiding principles for the provision, delivery and funding of healthcare provided to all community members. We propose a set of shared values and foundational beliefs to be applied in all communities using the Elevate Health Market brand. Any community may join, contribute to, and benefit from Elevate Health Markets, regardless of their geography, politics, religion, or culture, as long as they adhere to these core principles.

Once all Members of the community are aligned, in Chapter 5, we introduce the patient-caregiver relationship as the essential healthcare service. We then establish a transparent market infrastructure leveraging Web3 and AI technology in Chapter 6. Once these basic concepts are established, we use Chapter 7 to introduce the entrepreneurs, leaders, and product developers under the term "Builders." They represent all the valuable contributors to health markets that are not direct Caregivers themselves.

In Chapter 8, we provide a roadmap for establishing public health systems that protect and serve the entire population in the absence of a central authority, such as the government or employer. The manual section of the book concludes with Chapter 9, which describes Jim Collins' Flywheel concept and illustrates how to fuel the assembly of all these components into a functioning, self-sustaining market, leveraging reimbursement from existing healthcare markets. Over the next 25 years, we anticipate a surge in independent communities seeking to provide healthcare to their local communities. These future users of the Elevate Health manual will benefit from all other Elevate Health communities as they themselves begin to contribute to the overall movement.

Why Now? The Opportunity of Historical Cycles

We stand at a unique moment in history. Every 80-100 years, our global society experiences fundamental transformation—what historian Neil Howe calls "Fourth Turnings" or generational cycles. The last such transformation occurred after World War II, creating the modern healthcare system we know today. Over the next 25 years, we are expected to experience the next great turning, projected to culminate around 2050. This represents a once-in-a-lifetime opportunity to design healthcare systems for the next century, learning from the successes and failures of the current cycle while harnessing three powerful waves of technological innovation.

Our Shared Values

While we welcome diverse approaches to implementing healthcare solutions, Elevate Health unites around three non-negotiable values:

1. **Health is a Human Right:** Everyone deserves access to quality healthcare, regardless of their background or circumstances.
2. **Sustainable Funding and Allocation:** We must invest in our healthcare system for the long term, ensuring equitable access for current and future generations.
3. **Aligned Incentives and Innovation:** We must foster collaboration and innovation to optimize resources and deliver the best possible care.

These values aren't political positions—they're practical necessities for building healthcare systems that actually work for human beings rather than extracting wealth from their suffering.

The Elevate Health Vision

Imagine a marketplace where everyone has access to quality care, regardless of their background or circumstances. A system where we invest wisely in long-term solutions, ensuring equitable access for generations to come. A system driven by collaboration and innovation, optimizing resources to deliver the best possible care. We expect – and encourage – diverse opinions on the best way to implement and regulate healthcare. However, if we can agree on these shared values, our society will improve human health more rapidly and fairly over the next 25 years.

While we acknowledge the existing healthcare system and its commitments to the Boomer generation, we believe a parallel path must be forged. We envision a new, complementary healthcare market, built from the ground up to be ready for 2050. This isn't about dismantling what's in place; it's about creating a system that's independent, resilient, and adaptable to the changing landscape while remaining compatible with existing systems where possible. Think of it like developing a new high-speed rail network alongside existing highways. Both serve transportation needs, but the high-speed rail offers a fundamentally different approach to travel speed and efficiency. This is the kind of transformative change we envision for healthcare.

Overview of the Book

The Elevate Health 2050 book comprises ten chapters, divided into three sections. In the first section, we outline the cyclical nature of our global society and the opportunity to learn from the experience of the current cycle, preparing for the incredible technological capabilities that will emerge as we begin a new one.

<u>Section: Cycles of Human Society</u>
Chapter 1: Opportunity
Chapter 2: Three Waves of Innovation
Chapter 3: Two Great Health Unlocks

In the second section, we describe the foundational and structural components necessary to assemble an Elevated Health market, independent of geography, politics, religion, and culture.

<u>Section: Foundations of an Elevated Health Market</u>
Chapter 4: Shared Values and Beliefs
Chapter 5: Patients and Caregivers
Chapter 6: Market Infrastructure
Chapter 7: Builders
Chapter 8: Public Health for the People
Chapter 9: Building the Elevate Health Market

In the third section, we illustrate the power of the three waves of innovation when elevated above petty squabbles to bring a positive impact on human lives.

Section: Illustration and Call to Action
Chapter 10: End Heart Disease by 2035

Bootstrapping Elevate Health 2050 Like an Open-Source Community

Imagine a future where the global health industry is not dominated by large corporations or bound by traditional structures, but instead operates as a thriving, collaborative ecosystem, much like an open-source community. This is the vision we hold for Elevate Health – a $10 trillion global health industry built from the ground up, fueled by innovation, patient-centricity, and the collective power of shared knowledge and resources. This "bootstrapping" approach emphasizes organic growth, self-reliance, and minimal external funding. Think of it as a grassroots movement within healthcare, where progress is driven by passionate individuals, healthcare providers, and entrepreneurs collaborating to create a more accessible, affordable, and effective healthcare system. This model prioritizes patient needs and caregiver well-being, fostering a sense of ownership and shared responsibility among all participants.

The success of open-source communities like WordPress provides a compelling template for Elevate Health. WordPress, the platform powering a significant portion of the internet, started with limited resources and a small group of dedicated individuals. Its growth was fueled by organic community involvement, collaborative development, and a shared passion for democratizing web publishing. This mirrors the vision for Elevate Health, where collective effort and shared resources can drive transformative change in healthcare. The WordPress story is one of evolution and adaptation. From its humble beginnings as a blogging platform, it has grown into a robust and versatile content management system. Key factors in its success include a relentless focus on user experience, a strong and supportive community, and a flexible architecture that allows for extensive customization. These elements are also crucial to the success of Elevate Health, ensuring that the future healthcare system is user-friendly, accessible, and adaptable to evolving needs and technologies.

The bootstrapping model, as demonstrated by WordPress and countless other open-source projects, has proven to be a powerful engine for innovation. By fostering a sense of shared ownership and purpose, Elevate Health can harness this same collaborative energy to address critical healthcare challenges. This requires careful consideration of key questions: How can we ensure our values are reflected in the future market? What incentives and structures will attract the brightest minds, particularly from the generations who will be most reliant on this system in 2050? By addressing these questions and embracing the principles of bootstrapping and open-source collaboration, we can pave the way for a truly transformative healthcare system that prioritizes patient well-being, accessibility, and affordability.

Process & Regulatory Innovation

The healthcare industry has often been slow to adopt new technologies, lagging behind other sectors in the use of cutting-edge tools and methodologies. This reluctance to change means that process innovation and regulatory innovation can often have a more significant impact than product innovations. While the latest medical devices or pharmaceuticals tend to grab headlines, it's the underlying processes and regulations that truly shape the delivery and accessibility of care. Think of it like a high-performance race car – even the most powerful engine won't reach its full potential without a finely tuned chassis and a clear track to race on.

To illustrate the power of process innovation, let's take a step back in time and look at the Ford Motor Company in the early 20th century. Henry Ford's Model T wasn't just a new car; it was a breakthrough in manufacturing. While gasoline engines already existed, Ford revolutionized the production process, creating an assembly line inspired by meatpacking plants. This dramatically reduced production time and costs, making the Model T affordable for the average American. By focusing on efficiency and standardization, Ford didn't just build a car; he built an industry, and in many ways, a new America.

The impact of the Model T was nothing short of revolutionary. It transformed the automobile from a luxury item into a practical necessity, changing how Americans lived and worked. Suddenly, people could travel further, commute to jobs, and explore the country like never before. This spurred the development of roads and infrastructure, created new jobs, and even fostered the growth of suburbs. Ford's process innovation democratized the automobile, paving the way for the modern car industry and shaping the world we live in today. It's a classic example of how optimizing the "how" can be just as impactful, if not more so, than the "what."

The power of process innovation isn't just a historical anecdote; it's backed by academic research. Scholars in fields such as innovation studies, strategic management, and operations management have long examined how process improvements can drive efficiency, reduce costs, and create competitive advantages. Thinkers like Clayton Christensen, known for his work on disruptive innovation, have shown how process innovations can enable disruption and challenge established players. Similarly, Henry Chesbrough's work on "Open Innovation" highlights how collaboration and external partnerships can lead to groundbreaking process improvements.

The key takeaway is that process and regulatory innovations often lay the groundwork for impactful product innovations. Just as Ford's assembly line enabled the success of the Model T, streamlining processes and optimizing regulations can unlock significant value in healthcare. By focusing on how care is delivered and the rules governing the industry, we can create a more efficient, affordable, and accessible healthcare system. This could mean anything from optimizing patient flow in hospitals to simplifying insurance claims processing – all with the goal of better serving patients and improving outcomes.

Regulatory innovation is also impactful. In a highly regulated industry like healthcare, new or updated regulations can have an outsized impact. Smart regulations can create new markets, level the playing field, and even drive societal change. Consider how safety and emissions standards shaped the auto industry, pushing manufacturers to innovate and create cleaner, safer vehicles. Similarly, in healthcare, regulations can incentivize the adoption of new technologies, promote data sharing, and ensure equitable access to care. We'll revisit this topic later when we discuss how HCA leveraged regulatory innovation to unlock the benefits of the for-profit model in healthcare. But for now, keep in mind that innovation isn't just about shiny new products; it's about optimizing the entire system to deliver better care.

A Patient-Centric Approach

One of the benefits of focusing on the vision of our ideal health market in 2050 is the freedom to design the most impactful key distinctions without the constraints of current market forces or entrenched incumbents. This allows us to reimagine healthcare delivery from the ground up. We have identified five key distinctions that will shape this future market, beginning with a primary focus on patients and caregivers.

Elevate Health is designed first and foremost to benefit its members, all of whom are patients. Our priority is providing healthcare services and tools that empower individuals to optimize their personal health and wellness. Central to this is the concept of a **Personal Wellness Coach**: a guide that helps members access the most valuable resources. Think of it as a personalized healthcare concierge, available to every member, that cuts through the noise and connects them with precisely what they need, when they need it. While the specifics of this core product are still in development, we envision a suite of services and tools that seamlessly integrate to provide comprehensive support for each individual's health journey.

The Personal Wellness Coach will be built around several core themes. Imagine a secure and encrypted repository for all your health information and records, readily accessible yet completely private. Picture a detailed history of your medications, labs, procedures, and every healthcare interaction, all meticulously tracked and organized. Envision a personal health context database where you can store your preferences, trusted physicians, and preferred news sources, ensuring that your unique context informs every interaction within the Elevate Health ecosystem. Finally, imagine a system that continuously monitors your health metrics, recording your actions, the tools and utilities you use, the procedures you undergo, and the caregivers you interact with, providing a comprehensive picture of your health evolution over time.

Called to Caregiving

While the primary focus of Elevate Health will be on individual patients, we envision a very high percentage of our Members will also elect to contribute their skills and abilities to serve as caregivers to others. For some, this will be obvious if they are a physician, nurse, or counselor. However, we will seek ways to involve as many members as possible in contributing care to others in the Elevate Health market. As we age, our personal networks naturally become smaller and less engaging. For many, this leads to a need for fulfillment, meaning, and human connection. Simultaneously, many of the care needs will not require advanced degrees and extensive training. To encourage and empower members to either strengthen their caregiving or become caregivers, Elevate Health plans to offer a second optional benefit: **Top of Calling** caregiver productivity add-on product. This tool will be built on top of the core Personal Wellness Coach, serving members based on their qualifications, capacity, and interests already stored in the members' health context database.

The "Top of Calling" brand is meant to signal the purpose of the tool. Many incumbent organizations have established programs designed to help providers practice at the "Top of their License." While this has been a useful concept, we believe it focuses too much on the transactional and billing aspects of healthcare. Most physicians, nurses, and other caregivers do not enter a career in healthcare to maximize billing or earn the most income. Instead, we will develop the Top of Calling caregiver productivity product to help members realize their true calling, in whatever form that may take.

The two products will be intrinsically linked together. It is our vision that the Personal Wellness Coach may help the Member discover opportunities to find meaning and purpose in providing care to other members. This will be true for licensed healthcare workers, as well as for non-traditional caregivers. For instance, members with personal experience navigating a cancer diagnosis may be willing to share experiences and provide empathic listening to other members earlier in their care journey.

Three Foundational Beliefs

Healthcare is emotionally charged and intensely personal. Our shared values will be helpful, but ultimately insufficient to engender trust and ensure alignment. To augment these values, we foster collaboration and promote transparency by including three Foundational Beliefs designed to drive positive change and shape a brighter future for healthcare markets.

Three Foundational beliefs:

#1: Upgrading outdated For-profit / Non-profit Categories
#2: Radical Market Transparency combined with Personal Data Privacy
#3: Race to the Top for Health

Public Health for the People

To truly elevate health for all, we must go beyond individual wellness and actively address public health needs. Imagine a future where sustainable and free public health utilities are readily available to everyone, regardless of their socioeconomic status. These utilities, supported by diverse funding sources, could offer essential services like health screenings, immunizations, and chronic disease management, ensuring no one is left behind. We envision a system where the private sector contributes its expertise and resources to enhance these public health initiatives. This could involve companies donating services like health education programs, technology solutions, or even employee volunteer time for community outreach. By fostering collaboration and innovation between for-profit and non-profit entities, we can accelerate progress and develop novel solutions to pressing public health challenges. This collaborative ecosystem would not only increase the visibility and impact of non-profit missions but also provide a platform for groundbreaking research and development through jointly funded initiatives.

Fair & Responsible Healthcare Resource Allocation

Achieving a truly equitable and effective healthcare system requires a careful and responsible approach to resource allocation. This means striking a delicate balance between incentivizing private sector involvement and safeguarding the independence and mission of non-profit organizations. While for-profit companies can bring valuable resources and innovation to the table, their participation must be guided by a genuine commitment to public health impact, not solely financial gain. Transparency and accountability are crucial in this model, with transparent reporting on all collaborations and contributions to maintain public trust. Perhaps most importantly, we need to acknowledge the significant infrastructural challenges that lie ahead.

Building the Elevate Health vision requires rethinking everything, from policy and regulation to reimbursement models, medical record-keeping, and claims processing. This is a monumental task, but one we believe is essential to creating a healthcare system that is truly fair, accessible, and sustainable for all.

Join Elevate Health

Elevate Health 2050 is more than just a book; it's a movement. We are building a community of individuals, organizations, and governments dedicated to creating a better future for healthcare. A future where the coming waves of innovation unlock unimaginable improvements in health and lifespan, a future where everyone has the opportunity to live a longer, healthier life. We invite you to join us: your experience, your drive, and your commitment to making a difference align perfectly with our mission. Become a member of the Elevate Health community, contribute your insights, and help us shape the future of healthcare. Together, we can build a lasting legacy for our grandchildren and future generations.

Chapter 1: Opportunity

Look, if you had one shot or one opportunity
To seize everything you ever wanted in one moment
Would you capture it, or just let it slip?

Eminem

Each of us gets one opportunity during our 100-year maximum lifespan to shape the future direction of human society. We mean this in a logistical sense, not a philosophical one. In this chapter, we will discuss specifically why this single point in time exists and why the next great change will occur before 2050. The last time such an opportunity to shape society occurred, we lacked the perspective to understand that the opportunity was coming. Therefore, no one was prepared. Yet, in the post-WWII reconstruction, the US and its allies were able to change human society in several positive ways.

Since our focus is on health, we will highlight two powerful and positive structural changes to global health that were created in this post-war period. The first was global public health organizations such as the World Health Organization. These bodies leveraged newly created communication technologies to extend best practices of public health research across the world. Second was the introduction of the for-profit business model in healthcare markets. During the war effort, governments recognized the benefits of partnerships with for-profit organizations. They allowed for the first time, collaboration between for-profit, non-profit, and government organizations to deliver healthcare services and pharmaceutical treatments to the growing population.

We will discuss these two foundational health innovations and illustrate how they led to dramatic improvements in the healthcare industry in Chapter 3. For now, the critical insight is that the last cycle is ending, and we observe diminishing returns from these ideas. The for-profit business model in healthcare has begun to be criticized, and global health organizations are declining in effectiveness. This book will not focus on repairing past innovations. No need. Our parents and grandparents did the best they could with their opportunities. Rather, we choose to learn from the past while preparing to seize our our once in a lifetime opportunity.

Elevating Our Perspective

The world around us moves in repeating cycles that we are all familiar with. The Earth rotates on its axis, creating the 24-hour, daily cycle of day & night. We also orbit in an elliptical path around the sun, causing the annual seasons of Spring, Summer, Fall & Winter. We learn about these cycles as children; they are so much a part of our lives that we barely think about them. This is because the short duration of the cycle, referred to in science as the cycle's "period," allows us to witness thousands of daily cycles, and depending on our age, tens of annual cycles.

Other cycles have longer periods and, therefore, are difficult to observe. Halley's Comet is a convenient example as it is reasonably well understood and has a cycle period of approximately the same length as the average human lifespan. This long period makes the comet relatively difficult to study. Halley's Comet is the only known short-period comet consistently visible to the naked eye from Earth. It appears every 72–80 years and was last visible from Earth in 1986. The next time we will have the opportunity to see Halley's comet will be in 2061. The comet's clear visibility from Earth allowed it to be observed and recorded by astronomers since at least 240 BC. However, it was not until 1705 that the English astronomer Edmond Halley understood that these appearances were reappearances of the same comet. As a result of this discovery, the comet is named after Halley.

In this chapter, we are going to examine two cycles with periods similar in length to the cycle of Halley's comet. This makes them somewhat difficult to observe as the period length causes the cycle to repeat only once in our lifetime. Early astronomers failed to realize the cyclic nature of Hailey's comet. Instead, they believed they were witnessing new comets for centuries each time the comet made its pass by Earth during its 72-80 year orbit around our sun. Halley's brilliance was in his ability to shift his mindset and perspective. He "elevated" his mindset to focus not on the specific occurrence of a comet in 1705, with its associated technical details, but instead on the recurring nature of the similar pattern occurring every 75 years over the course of ~2,000 years. This elevated perspective allowed Halley to make his breakthrough discovery and earn international recognition.

We have the same opportunity to elevate our mindset just as Halley did 300 years ago. It is challenging because the period of our cycles is also long enough that most humans will only experience one cycle during their lives. Yet, this is also the opportunity. By carefully examining the facts, we can gain insight that others don't yet have and use it to elevate health for the benefit of everyone in the next 80 to 100-year cycle.

Luckily, we are not tasked with discovering these cycles. Rather, we get to stand on he shoulders of two other well-documented researchers: Ray Dalio and Neil Howe. Both have written entire books on their subject, and we will not attempt to replicate their full work here. Rather, we summarize their findings, celebrate their insights, and focus on how this elevated point of view offers us a generational opportunity.

Debt & Political Order Cycles (Ray Dalio)

Ray Dalio, the founder of Bridgewater Associates, the world's largest hedge fund, is known for his self-proclaimed apolitical stance and over 50 years of experience as a global macro investor. Dalio possesses a unique lens through which he views the world. His concept of a currency and debt cycle is described in multiple books and public speeches.

Ray's professional life and hedge fund strategy have been to strive to understand long-term, historical patterns and cycles. He believes that while specific events may seem surprising, like Halley's comet, their underlying dynamics have often repeated in many previous cycles of history. Dalio developed a comprehensive framework called the "big cycle" of changing world orders. His research delves into the last 500 years of history, meticulously studying the rise and decline of leading empires and their corresponding reserve currencies, such as the Dutch, British, and US empires. Dalio estimates the period of these "big cycles" to be about 250 years, often punctuated by highly disruptive 10 to 20-year transition periods. A core tenet of his philosophy is that history, while never identical, tends to repeat in fundamental patterns.

Within these cycles, Ray identifies several key forces that perpetually drive the health and wealth of nations. Among the most relevant to our interest is the long-term debt cycle, which typically lasts about 80 years. In this recurring cycle, debt persistently rises relative to income until inherent limitations are reached. Closely coupled with this is the political order cycle. This cycle runs in parallel with the debt cycle and describes a phenomenon where increasing wealth and value gaps within a nation inevitably lead to greater conflict and eventually political disorder.

Applying his framework, Dalio has widely observed that the United States is facing a critical juncture within these interconnected cycles. He suggests that the US is approaching the end of boht the Debt and Political Order cycles. In the past, such ends to these cycles have resulted in profound changes in "domestic order," and equally profound shifts in the "world order." In his books and speeches, Ray draws many parallels between the present era and the turbulent 1930s, citing commonalities such as rising protectionism through tariffs, burgeoning national debt, and the unmistakable dynamic of a rising power directly challenging an existing global hegemon.

Dalio's primary financial concern revolves around the escalating debt situation, particularly the sustainability of government debt. He states that the government is "going to be in financial trouble" due to the unsustainable growth of its liabilities. He foresees a critical supply/demand problem in the bond market: the sheer volume of government debt being issued is expected to outstrip demand, partly because existing holders already have a high percentage of their portfolios in government bonds and due to evolving geopolitical considerations. Ray argues tha central banks will be forced into an unenviable choice: either dramatically raise interest rates, which would severely harm the economy and financial markets, or resort to printing vast amounts of money to purchase the debt, inevitably leading to currency devaluation and inflation. This dynamic, in Dalio's view, represents a clear "breaking down of the monetary order."

Beyond financial concerns, Dalio points to increasing internal conflict as a significant vulnerability for democracies in this stage. As the debt cycle progresses, he explains, it frequently leads to a widening chasm between the "haves" and "have-nots," creating larger wealth and values gaps. These disparities, he warns, "increasingly create greater and greater conflicts" between different societal groups. He characterizes this as a fundamental challenge to the "domestic order" and a potential "fight between the two" sides, referring to the rise of left and right populism. If these growing divisions are not managed effectively, Dalio suggests, they could tragically escalate to a "great civil war or a conflict."

Insights from Cycles of Debt & Political Order

One key lesson from these historical studies is the recurrence of patterns resulting from logical cause-and-effect relationships. These patterns are readily observable if we take the proper perspective and time horizon. Dalio’s research into the Dutch, British, and US reserve currency empires led to the development of the "big cycle" template. By translating historical findings into objective measurements and statistics for various indicators like education, inventiveness, economic output, and military strength, Dalio developed "archetypal models". Comparing the data from empires like the Dutch and British allowed him to see the composition of these cycles through numbers, which helps indicate what stage a country is in and anticipate future developments.

Specific patterns of decline observed in empires like the Dutch and British provide vital lessons. As countries become more successful, they often become more expensive and less competitive. The work ethic can change, as people enjoy more leisure and become accustomed to an easy life. In support of Howe's work, Dalio finds that values shift across generations, from those who fought for wealth and power to those who inherited it, making them less battle-hardened and more vulnerable. Financial bubbles tend to grow as the population becomes used to doing well and borrows money to bet on continued good times. Ultimately, this leverage gets too high, leading to financial crises where debt and debt service become unsustainable. Historically, this has often culminated in massive money printing and currency devaluation, as seen in the Dutch case after their defeat and inability to repay debts.

Additionally, Dalio provides detailed historical studies of the US in the 1930s and Germany's hyperinflation in the 1920s to emphasize the crucial lesson about managing debt crises. They demonstrate that severe economic challenges can be navigated effectively if policymakers grasp the dynamics and have the knowledge and authority to apply the appropriate levers, such as austerity, debt restructuring, and monetary printing. However, the consistency of human nature also means that similar political and social challenges in managing these cycles tend to repeat. One cannot fail to observe the concerning parallels of money printing, inflation, and currency devaluation in our markets today.

Cycles of World Culture (Neil Howe)

The concept of cyclical history, as articulated by Neil Howe and William Strauss in their book "The Fourth

Turning," offers another compelling framework to help us understand coming societal changes. Howe and Strauss argue that history unfolds in recurring cycles, each lasting roughly 80 to 100 years, a period they term a "saeculum." Within each saeculum are four distinct "turnings" – High, Awakening, Unraveling, and Crisis – each characterized by differentiated values, societal beliefs, and cultural norms. Each generation of children is born into a unique time in history.

Human generations are estimated to be 25 years in length. This is because women typically begin giving birth to their children, which of course is the next generation, in their late teens and early twenties. The authors, Howe & Strauss, observed that each generation is raised by the generation before them using a different parenting style than their parents. This approach to parenting and raising children is influenced by how they were raised as well as world events occurring during their teens when they were "coming of age." This pattern repeats with each successive generation. The children are shaped by their parents and by world events as they are maturing. Then the baton is passed, and a new, different generation is conceived, born, and shaped. This cyclical pattern, driven by the interplay of generational archetypes, has profound implications for understanding the evolution of various sectors, including healthcare.

Central to the Fourth Turning theory is the idea that history is not a linear progression but rather a series of recurring patterns. Howe and Strauss challenge the conventional view of history as a continuous march of progress, suggesting that societies experience periods of growth, introspection, fragmentation, and crisis in a predictable cycle. They contend that this cyclical pattern is driven by the interaction of four generational archetypes – Prophet, Nomad, Hero, and Artist – each born during a specific turning and carrying a distinct set of values and characteristics. As these generations mature and assume leadership roles, they shape society in accordance with their generational values, beliefs, and norms, perpetuating the cycle.

The four turnings represent four distinct phases within the 80-100 year saeculum. The First Turning, or High, is a period of societal rebuilding and consensus following a Crisis. The Second Turning, Awakening, is marked by a focus on individual and spiritual needs, challenging the established order. The Third Turning, Unraveling, sees a rise in individualism and a decline in social cohesion. Finally, the Fourth Turning, Crisis, is a period of upheaval and societal restructuring, often involving conflict and a redefinition of social values. Understanding these turnings is crucial for anticipating societal shifts and their impact on various sectors, including healthcare.

Insights from the Fourth Turning Framework

Applying Howe's Fourth Turning framework to healthcare provides valuable insights into the evolution of this industry. The current saeculum, which we might call the "US Empire I," began after World War II and has witnessed significant changes in all aspects of society, including healthcare. The post-war High Turning was a period of rebuilding. Key foundational institutions such as the World Health Organization (WHO) and the National Institutes of Health (NIH) were established, reflecting a growing emphasis on global health and scientific advancement. The Awakening of the 1960s and 70s shifted as expected to focus on individual and spiritual needs, challenging the established order. It was during this time that the US created social programs like Medicare and Medicaid, expanding access to care but also introducing the for-profit model into healthcare delivery.

The Unraveling period began in 1985 and witnessed rising healthcare costs, debates over healthcare reform, and technological advancements. In 2005, we entered the 4th Turning - Crisis. Adverse events, including Hurricane Katrina, the Great Financial Crisis, and the COVID pandemic, have unfortunately marked this period. On the healthcare front, we can observe increasing consolidation in the industry and growing concerns about healthcare disparities. The Fourth Turning framework suggests that this period will likely involve significant restructuring of the healthcare system, potentially leading to new models of care delivery and a re-evaluation of the role of for-profit entities in healthcare.

The establishment of the Centers for Medicare & Medicaid Services (CMS) in 1965 marked a pivotal moment in U.S. healthcare. CMS oversees two of the largest healthcare programs in the country, providing coverage to millions of Americans. The creation of CMS expanded access to care for vulnerable populations and significantly influenced the growth of the healthcare industry. However, it also introduced the for-profit model into healthcare delivery, raising questions about the balance between profit and patient care. Understanding the role of CMS is crucial for navigating the complexities of the U.S. healthcare system and anticipating future changes.

Overlaying significant healthcare changes onto the cyclical framework reveals how societal trends have shaped the industry. The post-war High saw a focus on hospital construction and the development of vaccines. The Awakening brought about social programs and the rise of for-profit healthcare. The Unraveling period was marked by technological advancements and debates over healthcare reform. The current Crisis is characterized by the COVID-19 pandemic, telehealth expansion, and a renewed focus on healthcare disparities. This analysis highlights the cyclical nature of healthcare reform and the ongoing tension between access, cost, and quality.

Howe's Fourth Turning theory, while not a crystal ball, offers a valuable lens for understanding historical patterns and anticipating potential future trends. It suggests that the coming Crisis may bring about significant upheaval in healthcare, potentially leading to new models of care delivery and a re-evaluation of the role of for-profit entities. To navigate this period, healthcare systems must prioritize equitable access, invest in the workforce, engage with communities, and uphold ethical decision-making principles.

Our Mission to Elevate Health

Howe and Dalio approach the subject from vastly diverse points of view, yet arrive at the same conclusion. We find their research and arguments compelling, if sobering. It's likely that through some combination of new generational perspectives or the extension of more and more debt, the US-led global world order that we have enjoyed over the last 75 years will end soon. However, these researchers are frustrating in that they fail to offer a viable path forward or recommend steps we can take to ameliorate the negative impacts on ourselves, our neighbors, or our country.

Elevate Health 2050 takes a different course. We accept that some combination of the arguments made by Howe and Dalio will cause a significant disruption to the global world order. However, we elect not to focus on the causes of this change nor predict the inciting incident. Nor do we attempt to forestall or halt the cycle. Rather, we take the optimistic view that although we cannot predict the exact nature of the crisis, humans will persevere. The sun will continue to rise in the East, ushering in a new world order for society. Yes, it may be difficult and scary. The last transition, World War II, certainly caused much human suffering and pain. We are not naive to this sober reality. Furthermore, we understand the new world order may be quite different than our current system. We accept this and leave it to others to debate these important but fraught issues.

The Elevate Health 2050 community starts with a key assumption that a new group will come to power and form a new world order, starting the cycle for the next 75-100 years. The purpose of this book is to serve as a framework for a health system or health market in the context of the new global world order. No matter what country, political party, religious belief, or government structure dominates the human experience for the next cycle, we aspire to define a simple yet powerful framework that future leaders may implement to elevate health and improve the lives of their people.

To achieve this ambitious mission, we must design a health market that is both highly effective and independent of such emotionally charged political and cultural debates. We do not take the opportunity lightly. It will be incredibly difficult to build such a framework. Yet we see an opportunity to improve global health for the next 100 years. Such a shift can only be accomplished in the transition period following whatever disruption and chaos occurs; there will arise one or several new world powers. This only happens once in any human lifetime, and we believe it will happen in the next 25 years. When the smoke clears and the dust settles, these new leaders will need a health system to care for their population. Elevate Health 2050 aspires to be the best option for the next generation of global leaders in the future. This is our mission and our opportunity.

Elevate Health above social and political debates:

We have a choice of how to prepare for the next 25 years before the new world order. It may be American Empire 2, or it may be some type of shared power arrangement. Our effort is to elevate health, no matter how the world governs itself in the next 4 generations. Debates around governance, tax policy, etc., should be held, but we are healthcare innovation experts - not political revolutionaries. I have spent my life bringing innovations out of the garage, coffee shop, or lab and finding profitable ways to deliver better care to as many people as possible at the lowest expense.

We seek to elevate health to a human right. No matter what flag flies, our vision is to come to a shared agreement as we assemble the next great world order. No matter what else, all people should agree to uphold three shared health values and three foundational beliefs.

Shared health Values:

- Health is a Human Right
- Sustainably funded across Generations
- Aligned Incentives and Innovation optimize resources

Foundational Beliefs:

- Redefining Providers as Public Health or High-Profit
- Radical Market Transparency and Personal Data Sovereignty
- Race to the Top for Health

We anticipate a broad debate and uncertainty surrounding the implementation, allocation, and regulation of health. However, if we share common values and beliefs, we believe our society will improve human health more quickly and fairly over the next 100 years.

Designing the Health Market of the Future

To understand the future of healthcare, we need to grasp the forces shaping our world. Economists often talk about the "Factors of Production" – Land, Labor, and Capital. Land, including natural resources, is mostly finite. This scarcity pushes us to use resources more efficiently or find alternatives. Labor, our human capital, is growing, which is both an asset and a challenge. A larger workforce and consumer base drive economic activity, but also increase the demand for resources, underscoring the need for sustainable practices. Finally, Capital encompasses the tools, machinery, and infrastructure that boost productivity. Investing in advanced medical equipment and digital health infrastructure, for instance, is crucial for a more efficient and effective healthcare system.

These factors operate within a global market framework where a growing global economy, measured by GDP, constantly pushes against the limits of our planet's resources. This tension fuels innovation – the drive to develop new technologies like renewable energy, adopt new business models like the circular economy, and implement new regulations like carbon pricing. Sustainability becomes paramount, requiring us to decouple economic growth from environmental damage. Think of it as a business needing to find ways to increase profits while simultaneously reducing its carbon footprint. Technology plays a vital role, enabling us to use resources more efficiently, discover substitutes, and lessen our environmental impact. However, even with sufficient resources globally, unequal distribution can create scarcity and conflict, highlighting the need for fair access to healthcare.

The challenge of inclusive growth is central to this discussion. Economic growth doesn't automatically lift everyone equally. Often, the benefits concentrate among the already wealthy, leaving marginalized communities behind. Limited access to education, healthcare, and economic opportunities can trap people in cycles of poverty, preventing them from fully participating in and benefiting from economic growth. Furthermore, the environmental costs of growth often disproportionately impact vulnerable populations who rely more directly on natural resources. Imagine a factory polluting a local water source – the impact is felt most acutely by those who live nearby and depend on that water.

To address these challenges and proactively shape a better future for healthcare, we introduce "Elevate Health." This initiative envisions the ideal healthcare market for 2050, driven by innovation in all its forms. Innovation is about unlocking new possibilities – whether it's discovering new technologies, developing new business models, or creating new social and economic systems.

Vision for 2050

By focusing on 2050 and working backward, we liberate ourselves from the constraints of the current system and embrace truly innovative thinking. It's like designing a new golf course without being limited by the existing terrain – our community can create something truly unique and optimized for the future.

This future healthcare market is both proactive and preventive, and seamless and accessible. Proactive and preventive care emphasizes wellness, optimizing health and well-being throughout life. AI-powered systems analyze individual risk factors and recommend personalized prevention strategies, while incentives encourage healthy choices. Imagine a smartwatch that not only tracks your activity but also provides personalized feedback and rewards for healthy behaviors. Seamless and accessible care eliminates waiting rooms, delivering care when and where it's needed through telemedicine, mobile clinics, and home health technologies. Integrated data ensures all health records are easily accessible and shared between providers, breaking down information silos. And, crucially, affordable, universal access to quality healthcare becomes a fundamental right, regardless of income or location.

This vision also prioritizes a human-centered and empowering approach, while embracing technological advancements. Care is personalized, compassionate, and respectful of individual needs and preferences. Patients become active participants in their care, empowered by clear information and support. Healthcare adopts a holistic approach, addressing the whole person, including physical, mental, and social well-being. This human-centric approach is interwoven with cutting-edge technologies like Web3, biotechnology, and AI, enabling personalized medicine, secure data sharing, and predictive analytics.

Finally, this future market is sustainable and equitable, built with backward compatibility in mind. A focus on prevention reduces the need for costly treatments and lessens the environmental impact of healthcare. Equitable access ensures everyone benefits from advances in healthcare, regardless of their background or location. Healthcare systems operate in an environmentally sustainable manner, minimizing their ecological footprint. To achieve this, a phased implementation introduces new technologies and models gradually, ensuring continuity of care. Payment and reimbursement models reward value and outcomes, aligning incentives with patient well-being. Public-private partnerships leverage the strengths of both sectors to drive innovation and accessibility. At the same time, systems for education and training will be needed to prepare the healthcare workforce for the evolving landscape of care delivery.

Elevate Health Market

The Elevate Health market is designed to maximize human quality of life. Its core principles are values-driven, prioritizing health as a human right, sustainable funding, continuous innovation, and aligned incentives. It's open and inclusive, welcoming diverse stakeholders, from individuals and organizations to governments. Critically, it focuses on backward compatibility, bridging the gap between the current system and the 2050 vision.

On the regulatory front, Elevate Health advocates for policies that promote data interoperability, patient data ownership, and telehealth adoption. It collaborates with regulators to establish clear guidelines and standards for AI and Web3 applications in healthcare, ensuring ethical and responsible use. Within the Elevate Health community, a self-regulatory framework further reinforces these ethical practices.

Types of Innovation

Product and technical innovation can create new jobs and industries, improve access to essential services, and lead to more sustainable practices. Think of telemedicine as expanding access to healthcare in rural areas. Process innovation can create new markets and promote more inclusive workplaces, like streamlining patient intake processes to reduce wait times and improve patient satisfaction. Regulatory innovation can level the playing field, encourage competition, and address social and environmental issues, ensuring that growth is sustainable and benefits all members of society. In essence, innovation is about creating a future where everyone has the opportunity to thrive.

Elevate Health recognizes the interconnectedness of technological, process, and regulatory innovation. Technological innovation encompasses AI, LLMs, Web3, personalized medicine, and more. Process innovation focuses on value-based care, patient-centric approaches, and tools that empower healthcare providers. Regulatory innovation drives data interoperability, telehealth adoption, and ethical AI guidelines. It's important to acknowledge that healthcare has often been a late adopter of technology. This means process and regulatory innovation can be even more impactful than product innovations in driving meaningful change.

Summary

The Elevate Health 2050 vision aspires to proactively shape the future of healthcare. It's forward-thinking, values-driven, and focused on aligning incentives with public health goals. Being open and inclusive fosters innovation and ensures the system meets the needs of all. Its emphasis on Web3 and AI for infrastructure and personalized care positions it to revolutionize healthcare delivery. Elevate Health is not just a vision; it's a call to action, inviting you to join a community dedicated to building a healthier future for all.

Chapter 2: Three Waves of The Intelligence Age

Any sufficiently advanced technology is indistinguish able from magic.

Arthur C. Clarke

The world around us is changing fast. Artificial Intelligence or AI gets most of the attention, but Elevate Health is tracking three waves of technical innovation that will lead us into the Intelligence Age. These technologies will drive incredible new capabilities and new risks. In this chapter, we describe expected advanced capabilities from three distinct areas: AI, Web3, and Biotech. Each of these emerging technologies is powerful, independent of the others. Yet we argue they will converge and comingle, leading to exponential growth in capabilities and complex feedback loops with unexpected outcomes. Elevate Health does not attempt to predict specific details or timelines. There are many other sources for such predictions, and we assert that these details are NOT important to our mission. Rather, our focus is to understand how these powerful waves of innovation will bring new capabilities and new risks to healthcare markets and public health.

AI Capabilities in 2050

Early AI excelled at tasks like identifying objects in images or categorizing text, essentially recognizing patterns within existing data. However, exponential growth in computational power, coupled with new algorithms and vast amounts of data, has propelled AI into an era where it can create entirely new content. This leap means AI is no longer just processing data related to the world around it. Instead, it is also imagining and envisioning what the world could be, mimicking human creativity and expanding its utility. To estimate AI capabilities twenty-five years in the future, we have attempted to use an intentionally conservative model for the growth in AI capabilities over this time. We assume linear growth of AI over the next 10 years and then a deteriorating rate of growth in the subsequent 15 years. We understand that current AI models are accelerating in their capacity, but believe it’s more conservative to model flat or declining growth rates. Using this conservative premise, we project capabilities that are likely to be part of everyday life on or before 2050.

Even with conservative projections, AI's capabilities by 2050 are expected to be dramatic. Without accelerating growth rates, we can anticipate AI achieving near-perfect generative abilities across various mediums: indistinguishable text, hyper-realistic images and videos, and highly functional code. This isn't science fiction; it's a logical extension of current trends, allowing AI to imitate reality with stunning fidelity. Imagine AI systems effortlessly drafting entire novels, producing cinematic-quality short films from a simple prompt, or writing complex software applications with minimal human intervention. These capabilities are profound and one of the reasons we feel so passionate about the need for a market system like Elevate Health 2050. By January 1, 2050, AI is expected to achieve:

- **Near-Perfect Generative Abilities:** Producing content (text, image, audio, video, code, 3D) virtually indistinguishable from human-created content, enabling mass personalization and automation of creative workflows.

- **Advanced Reasoning and Problem Solving**: Functioning as "Expert Systems on Steroids" within defined domains, offering unrivaled data analysis and enhancing scientific discovery in fields such as healthcare and materials science.

- **Perfect Language and Communication:** Offering real-time, seamless translation; human-like, context-aware, and emotionally intelligent conversations; and automated report generation and summarization.

- **Ubiquitous Autonomy and Control:** Leading to sophisticated robotics, automated infrastructure (e.g., smart grids, supply chains), and self-managing software systems operating with minimal human oversight.

The world is rapidly moving beyond the Information Age into what many are now calling the Intelligence Age. This profound shift isn't merely about processing vast amounts of data; it's about systems that can learn, reason, and create, fundamentally altering how we interact with technology and each other. Just as the internet revolutionized access to information, AI is redefining what's possible, driving a new paradigm where intelligent automation and generative capabilities become central to our daily lives. This transition promises to unlock unprecedented levels of productivity and innovation across every sector.

Implications for Work & Society

Such powerful AI systems will lead to massive economic restructuring and redefinition of "work." Many jobs will be impacted, including information, management, and creative careers. Society will face information overload and an authenticity crisis due to the convincing nature of AI-generated content. Profound ethical and societal pressures will arise concerning wealth distribution, human meaning, and purpose. Geopolitical shifts are also likely, as nations effectively deploying AI gain strategic advantages.

One of the best books on this subject is Mustafa Suleyman's *The Coming Wave*. It explores the central dilemma that humanity's future both depends on the progress enabled by AI and is also imperiled by it. He focuses on the "containment problem," defined as the challenge of managing AI's rapid proliferation. Suleyman shares our views on the growth in AI capabilities, suggesting that AI will enable near-perfect content generation and multi-time horizon planning for complex tasks. He expects AI to amplify both the best and the worst in humanity. Suleyman is optimistic about the potential for AI to drive improvements in healthcare through the discovery of new knowledge and new science in medicine. However, he also describes multiple concerns, including misinformation, deepfakes, societal fragility, and inequalities in wealth and political power. Suleyman proposes to contain AI systems with "good functioning governance and oversight." He advocates for leading AI companies to undergo an audit and independent scrutiny and for governments to build technology and appoint technical oversight experts actively. The Coming Wave provides a great description of the future potential and peril of AI systems. However, we view his recommendations for containment as naive and inadequate.

Impact on Healthcare

Artificial intelligence is poised to deliver a fundamentally upgraded healthcare market, reshaping how we approach health and wellness. This transformative power stems from AI's unparalleled ability to accelerate the discovery of new medical knowledge, invent groundbreaking scientific solutions, and optimize existing healthcare systems with precision. We can expect more accurate diagnostics, personalized care plans, and entirely new treatments. AI promises not incremental gains, but a foundational shift towards more effective, data-driven care. By 2050, we expect high-quality, personalized health and wellness support to become universally accessible. Imagine a world where every individual has a dedicated personal health & wellness coach, serving simultaneously as a nurse, scientific advisor, research assistant, personal trainer, tutor, motivation coach, and confidant. AI's capacity to synthesize vast amounts of information and adapt to each individual's needs means expert guidance, typically reserved for a few, can now be scaled to empower everyone, democratizing access to sophisticated health management tools.

The practical application of such personal AI is already emerging. Platforms like Inflection AI's "Pi," which Mustafa Suleyman founded, exemplify this vision. The product is a chat-based LLM like many others, but Pi is designed to be a more empathetic AI tool with both exceptional emotional intelligence (EQ) for social support and robust intellectual capabilities (IQ) for factual accuracy. This blend of emotional understanding and actionable intelligence is especially important as we begin to use the technology in healthcare. At Elevate Health, we are building on this promise, recognizing that our community members are both patients and often compassionate caregivers. Our free EH Personal Health AI-Coach is a core member benefit, a tool designed to connect every patient to the most valuable community resources for their personal health and wellness journey. Furthermore, over 75% of our members choose to contribute their natural skills as caregivers. We offer these caregivers the Top of Calling caregiver productivity tool. This second AI companion empowers caregivers by maximizing their time and energy, enabling them to focus on their true calling: providing empathic support. It aligns perfectly with AI's potential to foster radical abundance and personalized well-being within a supportive community.

The Intelligence Age:

Our three innovation waves: AI, Web3, and Biotech, are already impacting health and healthcare. We describe these new technologies as waves because they will build, crest, and flow across our entire industry. The innovation waves will advance on an exponentially accelerating trajectory over the next 25 years. By 2050, the convergence of advanced capabilities from the three waves of AI, Web3, and Biotech innovation will democratize intelligence, empowering individuals and small teams. These new capabilities will trigger a societal shift from the Information Age to the Intelligence Age. To be clear, we are not the first to use this term. Sam Altman, CEO of OpenAI, first coined the "Intelligence Age" last in September 2024.

This new reality is still coming into focus, but Elevate Health believes the effects on healthcare markets will be significant and widespread. The Intelligence Age will lead to a growth in society's capabilities to deliver free or inexpensive products and services at a rate much faster than people, investors, existing companies, doctors, and patients understand, leading to an unrealized customer surplus. Five significant changes will characterize this new Intelligence Age:

1. **Re-evaluation of Values and Beliefs:** The transformative potential of AI, Web3, and BioTech will challenge fundamental assumptions about human work, creativity, and purpose, leading to a widespread re-evaluation of societal values and beliefs.

2. **Exploration of Novel Governance Models:** The unprecedented new capabilities will necessitate the exploration of new governance frameworks and

resource allocation models to ensure equitable distribution of benefits and mitigate potential risks.

3. **Human-AI Symbiosis:** Humans and AI agents will form deeply integrated partnerships, built on Web3 technologies and leveraging the unique strengths of each. AI agents will excel in tasks requiring rapid processing, vast knowledge bases, and complex computations, while humans will contribute critical thinking, creativity, ethical judgment, and emotional intelligence.

4. **Rise of the "Orchestrator" role in society:** In the Intelligence Age, humans will increasingly adopt the role of Orchestrator, leveraging a deep understanding of multiple interconnected domains. This broad perspective will enable humans to effectively collaborate with and leverage the specialized knowledge of AI tools, new infrastructure powered by Web3 technologies, and BioTech capabilities to develop and implement novel solutions to complex problems.

5. **Transformation of Healthcare:** The Intelligence Age will see a profound shift in healthcare and public health, with new AI, Web3, and BioTech tools playing a central role in diagnostics, treatment planning, drug discovery, and personalized medicine. This will require a reimagining of healthcare systems and professional roles to optimize patient care.

In the long run, these changes will be incredibly positive. Yet we expect the transition period to be chaotic and difficult. There will be broad debate and uncertainty over issues related to how best to implement, allocate, and regulate health in this new environment. Our goal is not to engage in political and social debates. Instead, we seek to elevate healthcare and public health as a set of shared values and foundational beliefs. If successful, we will establish health and healthcare as a human right. Our community will align on core values and foundational beliefs, enabling individuals, organizations, and states to implement and allocate healthcare in accordance with a diverse set of political and social policies. This combination of strict value alignment coupled with the freedom to pursue diverse health policy allocation strategies will improve human health faster and more fairly in the Elevate Health Markets of 2050.

Build Away from "the Frontier"

The media and technology communities have been focused on frontier LLMs in the pursuit of incredible new capabilities and artificial general intelligence (AGI). While this is intellectually interesting and worth following, it is not applicable in healthcare markets. The frontier models are, by definition, untested and also expensive. In healthcare, we are not early adopters of new technology. The healthcare industry has been systematically late to adopt technology, relative to other markets such as finance, manufacturing, and consumer products. This occurs due to the combination of two market factors: (1) an intense focus on patient safety, combined with (2) the high levels of government regulation. We do not expect the late adoption trend to change by 2050. Therefore, Elevate Health takes the unusual perspective of not focusing on the frontiers of AI research. Instead, our focus is on AI tools and models that are one or two versions behind the most cutting-edge models. The benefit of this election is that these “trailing” AI Tools are better understood, more reliable, and less expensive.

Elevate Health will build future health markets with reliable, repeatable capabilities of AI technologies. We expect these AI tools to be widely available as open source and relatively inexpensive to implement. Advancements in AI over the last 3 years have increased the potential for healthcare products and services far beyond those available in the market today. Over the coming 25 years, this gap between what is possible using established technology and what is offered in the market will continue to widen. For these reasons, there is no need to use expensive or untested models. Instead, Elevate Health will develop the infrastructure, tools, and context to help our three core member types: Builders, Caregivers, and Patients, convert this technical potential to actual health and wellness benefits.

Wave Theory of Technology Impact:

AI, Web3, and Biotech are each emerging as stand-alone impactful forces, possessing the capacity to reshape our economy and society. However, Elevate Health proposes that the full impact of these technologies cannot be appreciated by solely studying them independently. Rather, we must assess the many ways in which these technologies actively influence one another, much like waves of water at the beach. We refer to this as the "wave theory of technology impact" to distinguish it from traditional linear assessments of technological impact. In this chapter, we first assess each of the 3 waves as stand-alone technologies. Then we end the chapter by describing the dynamic and interactive nature of these technologies to evaluate the full combined impact.

Wave 1: Artificial Intelligence Foundation & Catalyst

Artificial Intelligence(AI) has exploded into our everyday culture and continuous news cycle. However, for our purposes, it is important to start by clearly defining what we mean by the term AI. The Elevate Health community defines Artificial Intelligence or AI as the capability of computer systems to perform tasks typically associated with human intelligence, such as learning, reasoning, problem-solving, perception, and decision-making. We view AI as a continuously evolving set of technology and computer systems designed to deliver intelligence, reasoning, problem-solving, writing, and decision-making at skill and quality levels approaching, equal and exceeding human-level performance. Behind these AI technologies, tools and products is a large field of research striving to develop ever-better methods, algorithms, software, and hardware that enable computers and other machines to perceive their environment and use learning and intelligence to take actions and achieve goals.

Powerful AI, as described by the CEO of Anthropic, Dario Amodei, in his essay, Machines of Loving Grace, provides a vision of what we can expect in the next 3-5 years. Of course, this is much faster than we are projecting, but we continue to attempt to be conservative in our projections. In terms of pure intelligence, the *Powerful AI* will be more intelligent than a Nobel Prize winner across most relevant fields, including biology, programming, math, engineering, and writing. This means it can prove unsolved mathematical theorems, write excellent novels, and write complex software code from scratch. Yet, in addition to just being smart, this future *Powerful AI* will be given interfaces to complete work projects through email, text, and SaaS tools such as Zoom, Slack, Teams, and Asana. Using these tools, the *Powerful AI* will be able to accomplish work projects similar to those that a human can achieve when working virtually. It will engage in all actions, communications, or remote operations enabled by this interface, including taking actions on the internet, taking or giving directions to humans, ordering materials, directing experiments, watching videos, making videos, and so on. The *Powerful AI*, does not just passively answer questions; rather, it can be given tasks that take hours, days, or weeks to complete, and then goes off and does those tasks autonomously, in the way a smart employee would, asking for clarification as necessary.

The potential for AI to transform the way we live, work, and play is significant. As AI products improve, they will increase efficiency, accuracy, and productivity across every sector, including healthcare, while enhancing customer experiences. AI-powered products already solve complex problems and make our daily lives more convenient. Additionally, these technologies are increasing in capability incredibly fast while simultaneously decreasing in cost. However, the rapid advancement of AI also presents significant challenges and ethical considerations. As the AI wave ushers in an era of unprecedented information overload, it will challenge our ability to discern truth amidst increasingly convincing AI-generated fake content. Deepfakes will pose serious threats, enabling fraud and even malicious acts like revenge pornography, eroding trust at a fundamental level. Beyond these intentional harms, AI's unchecked proliferation could trigger massive economic restructuring, leading to significant job displacement and potentially exacerbating societal inequalities if the wealthiest race away the fastest. There is real concern about the potential for widespread unemployment as many jobs become replaceable by machinery and robots. Consider a hypothetical scenario where an AI-driven system automates a significant portion of diagnostic radiology, leading to widespread job losses for human radiologists. While efficiency might increase, the long-term consequences could include a decline in human expertise, a widening gap between those who adapt quickly and those who don't, and a more fragile healthcare workforce susceptible to systemic shocks.

Issues such as privacy, security, and job displacement are critical challenges that accompany the AI innovation wave. These issues are of particular concern from a health and well-being perspective. Both actual job losses and anxiety over possible future job insecurity lead to behavioral health needs. Furthermore, personal health data must be secured and protected. The dual nature of AI—offering immense benefits while posing significant challenges—suggests it is not uniformly positive or negative but presents complex internal dynamics. This inherent duality means AI is a force with both constructive and potentially disruptive potential. When this "wave" interacts with Web3 and BioTech, its complexities will influence the overall emergent outcome, potentially amplifying both benefits and risks in unforeseen ways. Ensuring AI remains a net positive force necessitates investment in research and development, alongside the creation of robust policies and regulations to promote its responsible use.

The rapid advancement and broad applicability of AI across diverse domains position it as an accelerant for the other technological waves. In June 2025, the World Economic Forum published its *Technology Convergence Report*, which describes AI as a "unique interlocutor for integrating, enhancing, and embedding across all other technology domains" due to its dynamic breadth of subcomponents and layered maturity landscape. This observation suggests that AI is not merely a standalone wave; rather, it fundamentally alters the growth trajectory or the very nature of other technology waves as they propagate and interact. The pervasive influence and versatility of AI make it a critical, almost foundational, component in any convergence scenario, acting as an amplifier for the impacts of Web3 and BioTech.

Wave 2: Decentralization and Empowerment with Web3

Web3 is an abbreviation referencing the set of technologies enabling the third generation of the internet. Most internet researchers consider the internet or the "Web" as evolving over 3 stages. These stages are recognized using the version numbering system common in software development. Version 1 of the web, Web1, was the age of static webpages retrieved from servers through a browser. In this stage, content was created by a small number of centralized "experts" and published via the Web1 technologies. With the launches of Facebook in 2004, and YouTube in 2005, social media changed this basic architecture and became known as Web2. In this new version of the internet, the users themselves have become a very significant source of content. Everyone creates this user-generated content, but it is controlled and monetized by a small group of companies referred to as Big Tech. Importantly, the Web1 infrastructure did not disappear; instead, social media content was built on top of it. Web3 offers the next step in the democratization of media. It utilizes blockchain technologies to enable users to create content and control/monetize it themselves.

However, Web3 does not stop with the democratization of media. Instead, it can be used to develop an economy in which individuals are empowered to conduct business directly with one another without the need for central facilitating authorities. If realized, this offers the promise of a more effective and fair economy in which everyone has the chance to participate. In this way, Web3 provides the opportunity to impact society. It holds the potential to contribute to the development of a more just and equal society by empowering people and encouraging trust. The Web3 foundational focus is on creating and developing technology that manages the decentralization of industries and empowers individuals. It represents a fundamental shift in control and value distribution, potentially creating a "wave" that directly challenges existing centralized power structures in society and the digital economy. These ideals contrast with the current centralized Web2 paradigm, where large corporations control data and platforms. In this way, the Web3 technology wave is fundamentally disruptive to established norms, institutions, and power dynamics.

Chris Dixon's influential book, *Read Write Own*, offers a compelling framework for understanding the internet's evolution through three distinct eras, each defined by how users interact with and control online networks. The initial "Read Era" (Web1, roughly 1990-2003) saw the internet as a collection of open, permissionless protocol networks such as email and the early web. This phase empowered users to read or access information, fostering immense creativity as value accumulated at the network's best-known writers and builders. However, by the mid-2000s, the "Read-Write Era" (Web2, roughly 2004-2020) emerged, dominated by corporate networks such as Facebook and Google. Dixon posits that the internet is now entering its third act: the "Read-Write-Own Era" (Web3), powered by blockchain networks capable of democratizing ownership. These aren't just databases; they are a new type of computer that can make commitments, establishing inviolable rules in software that guarantee future behavior. This architecture facilitates shared ownership and decentralized governance, returning power and economic benefits to communities and individual users.

Key advantages of Web3 technologies for users include the revolutionary concept of digital ownership through "tokens." From a market perspective, Web3 networks enable users to leave a service and take their digital assets or audience with them. Web3 services also feature persistently lower fees to the platforms. This allows more of the value to be shared by creators and users, fostering many new contributors and robust competition. Additionally, Web3 technology is highly composable, allowing software components to be mixed and added together like Lego bricks. This enables driving innovation on top of existing structures, much like the success realized in open-source software projects.

Web3 technologies are still in the nascent stage of development and behind AI in terms of market readiness. The technology is developing, and we expect ongoing hurdles related to regulatory uncertainty, technical scalability, and the potential for new forms of digital inequality. The trustless nature of Web3 and its use of blockchain for data integrity, privacy, and decentralization position it as a critical enabling layer or infrastructure for other technological waves, particularly those dealing with sensitive data, such as healthcare applications. As Web3 technology matures, it will enable secure, yet open records that allow proper updates while preventing unauthorized use, ensuring data integrity, privacy, and decentralization. This suggests Web3 is not just a standalone wave but a potential enabling infrastructure component that allows other waves to propagate more securely and effectively.

The combination of Web3 and artificial intelligence will bring transformative changes in multiple fields, including healthcare. Web3 technologies directly address critical questions arising from AI's rapid development, such as content ownership, compensation for creators whose data trains AI models, and ensuring transparency and verifiable control over AI systems to counteract centralizing tendencies. Imagine a future where patients genuinely own their health data through privacy-preserving Web3 networks or tokens, similar to owning physical possessions. Concepts like self-sovereign identity in healthcare empower individuals to control access permissions to their medical records, fundamentally shifting agency from institutions back to the patient. Furthermore, Web3 enables innovative uses of token incentives in wellness, rewarding healthy behaviors like exercise or medication adherence, and bootstrapping community-owned health data cooperatives where individuals contribute de-identified data for research and earn rewards. Direct-to-consumer health services could bypass traditional intermediaries, leveraging blockchain's advantages to deliver more affordable, patient-centric care, offering a new path to solve current system inefficiencies.

Elevate Health believes Web3 technology will be very positive only when two key issues are resolved. First, the core technology is very complex and, therefore, subject to both honest errors and intentional fraud. We must leverage the power of AI to simplify the complex blockchain transactions, simplifying mass market adoption. Second, the Web3 innovation wave must be constrained by shared values and foundational beliefs. These act as guardrails, allowing the use of these powerful tools without significant societal friction or public dissent. The key impacts of Web3 include empowering individuals by granting them greater control over their data and enhancing privacy, as users own their data and decide how it is used, free from censorship or unauthorized sale to advertisers. This is especially important in health settings as personal health records, DNA sequences, and health decisions are intensely personal and must be protected.

Blockchain protocols can also be leveraged to make health data from electronic health records, wearables, and genomic tests truly composable like Lego bricks. This could mean a patient's comprehensive health data is securely shared and integrated across various applications—a diet app pulling from a genomic profile, a fitness tracker linking with a chronic disease management platform, or an AI-powered doctor's assistant accessing a full, multi-source medical history. This seamless integration promises personalized health insights and coordinated care, breaking down entrenched data silos. While AI can revolutionize diagnostics and personalized medicine, blockchain is crucial for addressing ethical and practical challenges: guaranteeing patient consent for AI training on sensitive data, establishing fair compensation for data contributions (especially for rare disease research), maintaining data integrity, and enabling decentralized AI models to be trained on distributed, privacy-preserving datasets. Ultimately, this paradigm shift, driven by patient control and compensation, can support human flourishing in an AI-driven healthcare world.

Wave 3: Reshaping Health, Environment, and Agriculture with Biotechnology

Biotechnology (Biotech) encompasses a range of areas, influencing fundamental health and wellness categories such as pharmaceuticals, diagnostics, and food. The biotech innovation wave holds incredible promise and inherent ethical, social, equity, and governance complexities. This makes the Biotech wave propagation and interaction with other technological waves particularly sensitive, albeit powerful.

Positive impacts of biotech are extensive. Specific health advancements include AI-powered drug discovery, which can identify potential drug candidates in a fraction of the time. One example of this is AlphaFold, an AI and Biotech system developed by Google, which has already had a significant impact by revolutionizing protein structure prediction. Biotech and AI will also combine to allow for the earlier diagnosis of disease by analyzing a combination of biometric data collected through wearable devices, medical images, and genetic data. Over the next 25 years, this will lead to personalized medicine, tailored to an individual's genetic makeup, lifestyle, and medical history. In addition to human health, agricultural biotechnology is also advancing quickly. One example is the biotech firm Ohala and its Boosted Breeding technology. This company has shown significant promise in enhancing potato yields and potentially revolutionizing potato farming. The Boosted Breeding technology allows for the creation of potatoes with all the genetic traits from both parent plants, instead of the usual half from each, resulting in higher yields and more uniform, disease-resistant seeds. This early example will be followed by hundreds more over the next several decades. Agricultural biotechnology will be a valuable tool for addressing climate change, improving global food security, and alleviating poverty through increased agricultural productivity.

Despite its vast potential, biotechnology also faces complex challenges and ethical dilemmas. Crucial questions of social equity arise regarding whether the benefits of biotechnology will be shared equally across different communities and countries, or if they might worsen existing inequalities. The broad range of ethical considerations, particularly concerning genetic modification and ensuring responsible innovation, is paramount to the prevention of improper use of these powerful tools. The profound and at times irreversible nature of its genetic interventions causes the Biotech wave to have a unique capacity for rapid and widespread societal transformation. Like Web3, Elevate Health believes that shared values and beliefs must constrain Biotech technology. By agreeing on a shared set of values and foundational beliefs about how to implement Biotech technologies, we can realize the benefits of these powerful technologies without significant public dissent or ethical concerns.

Illustration: Robinhood's On-Chain Revolution

Robinhood is taking an ambitious leap into the future of finance, embarking on a major initiative to rebuild its entire financial platform on crypto rails.1 This isn't just about offering Bitcoin and memecoins; it's about leveraging blockchain technology to provide "fundamental utility" through tokenized assets. A key focus is democratizing access to wealth-generating opportunities. Robinhood has already launched tokenized US stocks and ETFs in the EU, with plans to introduce thousands more by year-end.2 A particularly significant move is the tokenization of private company shares, such as those in SpaceX and OpenAI, making these typically inaccessible assets available to retail investors.3 As Robinhood CEO Vlad Tenev emphasizes, if institutional investors have access to a product, retail investors should too. This tokenization also enables 24/7/365 trading, eliminating the constraints of traditional market hours and addressing long-standing inequities in capital markets.4 The long-term vision is to bring the entire Robinhood ecosystem on-chain, including real estate and art, ultimately simplifying complex financial instruments and encouraging broader adoption of crypto rails for financial transactions.

The success of this partnership hinges on Arbitrum's strategic dual approach, which offers both a robust public chain (Arbitrum One) and a customizable stack (Arbitrum Orbit) for building custom chains. Robinhood initially utilized Arbitrum One's "deep liquid platform" for its tokenized stocks, allowing for an immediate launch.

However, the plan is to migrate to a proprietary Robinhood L2 built on Arbitrum's Orbit stack. This migration is seamless because it uses the "exact same software stack," ensuring continuity without needing to change contracts. The Orbit stack is appealing due to its unparalleled flexibility, allowing for custom gas tokens, alternative data availability layers, and specific ordering flows.5 Furthermore, Arbitrum's Stylus feature is a key differentiator, allowing developers to code in Rust, C++ and other languages, addressing the potential difficulty in finding Solidity developers.6 Arbitrum's business model for Orbit chains, which involves a 10% profit share paid to the Arbitrum DAO, aligns economic incentives with ecosystem growth, positioning Arbitrum as an ideal platform for institutional optionality and growth.

This partnership signals a fundamental shift toward "finance powered by crypto," where the traditional distinction between TradFi and DeFi becomes increasingly blurred. The long-term vision is that blockchain technology will serve as the backbone of the global financial system, enabling compliant and highly usable products. The goal is to abstract the technical complexity of the blockchain away from the end-user. Users will benefit from instant, 24/7 transactions without needing to understand the underlying protocol. For institutions like Robinhood, owning a chain allows them to internalize revenue from transaction fees and MEV (Maximal Extractable Value), transforming operating expenses into revenue. This shift toward on-chain finance and tokenization also offers significant societal benefits, democratizing wealth creation and providing global access to attractive US assets, particularly in regions with devaluing currencies.

Both Robinhood and Arbitrum are actively engaging with policymakers to shape a favorable regulatory environment for on-chain finance. Robinhood believes that the tokenization of public equities in the US can be achieved through "exemptive relief" from the SEC, similar to Reg ATS, rather than requiring new congressional action.7 They are also advocating for a "complete rethink of the accreditation rules" for private company tokenization, favoring "self-certification-based" approaches. The launch of perpetual futures in the EU was made possible by licenses, while US availability remains contingent on CFTC approval. The structure of the Arbitrum DAO, with its significant treasury and token holder authority, enables bold strategic decisions, leveraging funds specifically allocated for strategic partnerships to land deals like the one with Robinhood.

The Robinhood-Arbitrum partnership is a bellwether for the financial industry, signaling a future where on-chain finance becomes mainstream. As the Robinhood app, now renamed "Robin," expands its reach, crypto rails will increasingly power traditional financial services, often invisibly to the end-user. This collaboration is a significant step toward a future where "everything is on-chain," moving beyond simple Bitcoin and memecoins to a place where crypto provides fundamental utility and democratizes access to assets for a global retail audience. The partnership also underscores the importance of regulatory clarity and the evolution of blockchain infrastructure into sustainable, customizable, and interoperable business models.

Wave Theory: Pulling it all together

The wave analogy has been widely used to help explain significant technological and societal change. This is because the wave is both familiar and descriptive. We all have direct experience with waves of water at the beach.

This allows us to visualize how waves form, build strength, crest, crash, and then recede. Yet waves are also valuable in their capability to model dynamic, interactive, and non-linear relationships. Traditional analyses often treat technologies as independent variables, assessing their impacts in isolation. The wave analogy, by its very nature, compels a consideration of interaction, superposition, and interference, which are inherently dynamic and non-linear processes. The inherent complexity of this proposition necessitates a nuanced exploration of the wave analogy as a tool to help us understand the long-term societal impact. Just as physical waves can constructively or destructively interfere, the convergence of AI, Web3, and BioTech can lead to amplification or dampening of societal impacts.

Two types of Interference: Amplification and Dampening:

When these technologies align, their positive impacts can be significantly amplified. For example, AI-powered drug discovery combined with blockchain for secure clinical trial data has the potential to accelerate the development of personalized medicine. This, in turn, can lead to better patient outcomes across the population. Additionally,

Web3's decentralized identity solutions, combined with AI for verifying interactions, can build a more trustworthy and safe digital ecosystem, protecting users from misinformation. The ability to decentralize health data sources, giving users control while incentivizing data allocation for scientific research, creates a positive feedback loop for faster and more accurate scientific discovery. Conversely, misaligned or poorly managed convergence can lead to amplified negative consequences or unforeseen dampening effects. For instance, if AI-driven automation leads to widespread job displacement and Web3-enabled financial systems exacerbate existing digital divides by excluding those without access or literacy, the combined effect could deepen societal inequalities. Additionally, ethical concerns in biotechnology, particularly around genetic modification, could be amplified by AI's predictive power and data sharing if not governed responsibly, leading to societal backlash. Understanding these potential amplification and dampening effects is crucial for proactive governance and policy-making. The non-linear nature of these interactions means that interventions in one area can have cascading, unpredictable effects across the entire socio-technical system

Strategic Imperatives:

Navigating these converging technological waves requires a proactive and adaptive strategic approach from policymakers, investors, and the broader society as a whole. Elevate Health will work to foster interdisciplinary research that explores the intersections and synergistic potentials of AI, Web3, and Biotech, rather than focusing on them in silos. This includes funding initiatives for convergence platforms and cross-domain expertise. In addition to sponsoring research and study, we will work to develop adaptive governance and appropriate regulatory frameworks. We believe that traditional regulatory approaches will struggle to keep pace with these rapidly evolving technologies. New frameworks must be agile, anticipatory, and capable of addressing the complex ethical, social equity, and security implications that arise from technological convergence. This requires ongoing dialogue between technologists, ethicists, legal experts, and policymakers. Lastly, Elevate Health recognizes that the future impact of these converging technologies will be emergent and non-linear. To prepare for this, we plan to encourage strategic planning that incorporates complex system dynamics, identifies feedback loops, and builds resilient, adaptive systems designed to understand and respond to unforeseen societal turbulence.

Social and Cultural Medium:
The concept of a "medium" is crucial for understanding wave propagation and interaction. Unlike a physical fluid, the societal medium is characterized by active human agency, collective decision-making, and emergent behaviors that continuously reshape its properties. This means the innovation waves not only propagate through the medium but also actively transform it, creating complex feedback loops. For example, the adoption of Web3's decentralized identity solutions fundamentally alters the medium of digital trust and privacy, which in turn affects how AI and BioTech applications are perceived and integrated. The societal medium is dynamic, with human agency reshaping how these waves propagate and interact. Elevate Health aims to foster an active community shaped by shared values and foundational beliefs, which then serve as crucial guardrails to ensure the technologies serve humanity. Thus, Elevate Health views this medium as a dynamic, adaptive socio-technical system that shapes,

channels, and constrains the three innovation waves. The medium comprises three related initiatives:

- **Elevate Health Community:** We aspire to develop an active and outspoken community of people focused on shaping these powerful technological waves toward our shared values and foundational beliefs

- **Shared Values:** As we navigate uncertain times and attempt to constrain and channel these technological waves, Elevate Health calls on all individuals, communities, and nations to unite around a shared vision for health. We believe health to be a fundamental human right, and we must work together to create a healthcare system that is sustainable, equitable, and innovative.

- **Foundational Beliefs:** Aligning efforts around core values helps to connect and align our community, but it isn't enough. Elevate Health also holds Foundational Beliefs to help shape the market in a positive direction and drive positive change. This approach will foster trust between patients and

> healthcare providers, creating a foundation for a more collaborative and effective healthcare system. Ultimately, this will create a health market in 2050 that prioritizes patient needs and ethical, sustainable practices.

The three waves of innovation hold immense potential to amplify humanity's greatest strengths, yet they also risk magnifying our deepest flaws. The challenge of managing AI's rapid proliferation and widespread disruptive potential has been termed the containment problem. However, Elevate Health observes that we must not only contain the AI wave but also the Web3 and Biotech waves. While there are a few efforts underway to address this with governance and oversight, they are severely underfunded and unlikely to have much of an effect.

However, a fundamental gap in the containment logic remains: AI cannot be truly "contained" because, as a society, we currently lack a universally agreed-upon set of shared values and beliefs. Experts may grapple with technical safeguards and regulatory frameworks, but without a clear definition of what is "good" or "bad" within human ethical systems, AI cannot inherently differentiate between helping or harming. This absence of a collective moral compass prevents us from any chance of significant constraint on AI capabilities. We believe this leads to the conclusion that it is structurally impossible to constrain AI, and yet we must find some means to mitigate risks if we are to reap the benefits.

Elevate Health is committed to building future health markets where reliable, inexpensive AI tools unlock a customer surplus in health and wellness benefits. We believe our social and cultural medium both clearly define what is "good" or "bad" within the Elevate health ecosystem and establish a framework to shape these three very powerful waves of innovation for the benefit of the human experience. This vision necessitates more than just technological advancement; it requires a profound re-evaluation of human values and the exploration of novel governance models.

In this coming Intelligence Age, humanity's role shifts towards becoming an "Orchestrator," guiding AI's development and deployment. Society must not become a passive recipient of these technological waves, as occurred with social media. Rather, Elevate Health strives to intentionally foster shared values and beliefs to act as a "medium" shaping the development of AI, Web3, and Biotech products through an emergent system of aligned incentives and natural checks on power. In this way, Elevate Health will foster a community aligned around shared health values and foundational beliefs as crucial guardrails. Realizing our future potential hinges on effectively navigating the containment problem, not through top-down governance or regulation, but through an emergent and bottom-up collective societal effort.

Chapter 3: Two Great Healthcare Unlocks

Those who cannot remember the past are condemned to repeat it

-George Santayana

After World War II, the US emerged as the dominant global technological, economic, and military power. Not only did America avoid the devastating destruction of physical infrastructure that occurred in Europe and Japan, but it also ended the war with a demonstration of technical and military dominance through the use of two nuclear weapons. The period following, from 1945-1970, marked one of the most significant transformation periods in human history. As we learned in Chapter 1, Neil Howe refers to this period as the "High Turning." Technological, political, and social changes reshaped virtually every aspect of society and culture. This new world order was led by the US but encompassed the entire world. For ease of reference and to distinguish it from other time periods, we refer to this as the United States I or US I.

Two innovations in healthcare and public health stand out as particularly consequential, not merely for their immediate effects but for their lasting impact on healthcare and public health. This chapter explores these two specific post-WWII innovations and how they "unlocked" incredibly positive leaps forward in human health and wellness. First, the emergence of the for-profit business model in healthcare, and second, the development of global communications networks enabling centralized public health. While these innovations might appear unrelated, we argue that they were both products of the unique circumstances created by World War II and its aftermath. Furthermore, these two "unlocks" also worked in concert to fundamentally alter the trajectory of health in the US and worldwide. As discussed in Chapter 1, we believe there will be an opportunity for one or more similar foundational "unlocks" in the immediate aftermath of the upcoming crisis period. Our purpose in this chapter is to learn from the two great unlocks of the last cycle with an eye to how we can most effectively improve health in the next cycle.

Importantly, we must plan this work without knowledge of any details of the coming crisis, not to mention the resulting global leadership. We hope for a US-led free and democratic new world order in 2050, but we must prepare for all future possibilities and attempt to optimize human health, regardless of the flag under which we live.

Healthcare Pre-WWII:

To understand the transformative nature of these post-war innovations, it is essential first to examine the healthcare landscape that existed before World War II. In the US and much of the developed world, healthcare in the early 20th century was characterized by several key features that the war and the following US-led rebuilding process would dramatically alter.

Healthcare markets before 1942 were predominantly based on direct payment by individuals. People paid for their medical care in cash, with limited insurance coverage. This system, while straightforward and similar to other markets, created significant barriers to healthcare access for many, particularly during economic downturns such as the Great Depression. The charity care that was provided to the public was delivered primarily by religiously affiliated and government-funded hospitals. Religious institutions, particularly Catholic hospitals, accounted for over 50% of all care. Government-funded city hospitals, which received funding from city and county sources, helped to provide care to poor populations. Private hospitals, often founded by local doctors, existed at this time; however, they were typically small and catered to the wealthy.

There was little international cooperation related to health before World War II. During the late 19th and early 20th centuries, the term international health referred to efforts to control disease epidemics across national borders, with neighboring countries, rather than being truly global. Communication constraints, limited by telegraph, mail, and slow transportation, severely hampered attempts at coordinated international public health projects. World War II catalyzed change across multiple domains, creating conditions that would enable the two health-related great unlocks during the post-war "High period." The war necessitated massive government intervention in the economy, leading to policies that would have far-reaching consequences. Simultaneously, the technological demands of warfare accelerated developments in communications and other technologies that would later find civilian applications. The global nature of the conflict also highlighted the interconnectedness of nations and the need for international cooperation on an unprecedented scale.

1st Great Health Unlock: For-Profit Healthcare

The emergence of for-profit healthcare businesses as a significant force in the American healthcare system represents one of the most important structural changes in healthcare markets following WWII. This transformation was not the result of deliberate policy design but rather the unintended consequence of wartime economic controls that created conditions favorable to the development of employer-sponsored health insurance. This was followed by President Lyndon Johnson's Great Society initiatives in the 1960s, which added health coverage for the elderly and poor populations. These regulations and programs combined to enable the development of a robust for-profit healthcare market.

The Birth of Health Insurance

The first of three catalyzing factors leading to for-profit healthcare didn't emerge from careful policy design. Instead, it was a result of the unintended consequences of wartime economic controls and their subsequent removal. This seemingly minor historical detail fundamentally altered the American healthcare landscape, establishing the foundation for our modern employer-based system. The US market's unique feature of providing healthcare insurance through employers can be traced directly to a specific piece of wartime legislation: the Stabilization Act of 1942. This act was designed to combat wartime inflation by freezing wages and salaries in September 1942. However, it specifically excluded health insurance from government control. This created a loophole that employers used to attract and retain workers in the tight wartime labor markets. Unable to offer higher wages, employers began offering health insurance as a benefit, thereby circumventing the wage controls. This policy led to the replacement of the cash settlement market with the employer-based insured health markets we know today. Wage controls were repealed in December 1945, following the end of the war. This triggered a return to the use of wages as the primary recruiting tool. Health insurance was no longer the sole loophole to increase effective compensation. Employee-sponsored healthcare might have disappeared but for another important law.

The second catalyzing factor was the Taft-Hartley Act of 1947. This law was the first legislative action in which the US began to intentionally improve individual healthcare rights as a part of establishing a new world order. As discussed in Chapter 1, we expect these changes to society during the "High period," described by Neil Howe. The Taft-Hartley Act restricted the activities of unions and expanded employee rights. The act made health benefits a mandatory subject of collective bargaining between organized labor and employers. This health requirement was further solidified by a 1949 Supreme Court ruling that confirmed health benefits must be negotiated, effectively stripping employers of their option to decline to offer healthcare benefits. The Revenue Act of 1954 further entrenched this system by confirming the tax exemption for employer health benefits. This tax policy cemented the employer-based system as a permanent feature. Through these legislative actions, health benefits became a legal obligation of employers rather than a voluntary strategy.

The growth of employer-sponsored health insurance created pools of covered patients whose medical expenses were paid by one aggregate source. This development altered the health market by concentrating the buying power of many individual healthcare consumers into a few health insurance organizations. These new participants in the market came to be known by the nickname "payor," due to their primary role as bill payor. As health insurance evolved into a corporate obligation, the organizations delivering this service evolved as well. The payors' primary customer was the company providing health insurance to its employees. Payors were asked to aggregate all the employees in a group or "insured pool" in order to manage the future healthcare expenses as a liability to be minimized. Benefits to individual employees needed to meet legal requirements and be attractive enough to keep employees. Over time, payors became focused on mitigating risk and reducing the costs of health insurance.

This transformation in healthcare financing created the

economic conditions necessary for the development of large-scale, for-profit healthcare enterprises. As large numbers of employees gained health insurance, they provided an attractive market for motivated businesses to serve. Prior to this period, healthcare had been a local, sub-scale industry characterized by individual practitioners and charity-funded hospitals. The availability of insurance coverage for large numbers of patients changed the economic calculus of healthcare delivery, making it possible to achieve economies of scale with predictable revenue streams and attractive profit margins.

LBJ's Great Society: Healthcare for the Elderly and Poor:

While the Stabilization and Taft-Hartley Acts led to employer-sponsored health insurance, the third major catalyst for for-profit healthcare growth came with the creation of Medicare and Medicaid as a significant part of the Social Security Act of 1965. This law was passed at the peak of the High period in the US and dramatically expanded the number of Americans with health insurance coverage. Medicare was established to provide healthcare insurance to all US citizens after they retire. Since workers already had coverage, this filled the void in healthcare after people stopped working. Lastly, non-working individuals, especially children and the poor, received coverage under Medicaid. In July 1965, President Johnson signed the bill and gave a speech about healthcare benefits as a key part of his Great Society. Below is an excerpt from the President's comments.

> *No longer will older Americans be denied the healing miracle of modern medicine. No longer will illness crush and destroy the savings that they have so carefully put away over a lifetime so that they might enjoy dignity in their later years. No longer will young families see their own incomes, and their own hopes, eaten away simply because they are carrying out their deep moral obligations to their parents, and to their uncles, and their aunts.*

- *P*
r
e
s
i
d
e

nt Lyndon B. Johnson

As the new legislation was being drafted, two businessmen from Nashville, TN, traveled to Washington to lobby Congress to modify the Social Security Act. Jack Massey and Tom Frist successfully added the ability for the government to reimburse both for-profit and non-profit healthcare providers for services. Because the federal government did not want to become involved in healthcare decisions made by doctors and to simplify the administrative process, Medicare and Medicaid established the policy of reimbursing healthcare providers at a rate equal to their cost plus a 30% additional margin. The significance of this development cannot be overstated. Medicare and Medicaid not only expanded coverage to previously uninsured populations (the elderly and the poor, respectively) but also established standardized payment mechanisms that reduced the financial risk associated with providing healthcare services. This standardization and risk reduction made healthcare an attractive market for investment.

With most Americans covered for healthcare services either by their employer or through Medicare and Medicaid, the US healthcare market became attractive and primed for growth. Many existing charitable hospitals expanded, and for-profit businesses entered the market. In 1967, Massey and Frist established the Hospital Corporation of America, known today as HCA, Inc. By 1971, there were 38 for-profit hospital chains in the US. The emergence and growth of for-profit healthcare led to increased capital investment in the sector and contributed to attracting talent to the healthcare workforce. Overall, this growth in the healthcare industry led to improvements across every aspect of the market.

2nd Great Health Unlock: Global Public Health

The second transformative innovation was the development of global communications technologies that enabled centralized planning and coordination of public health initiatives across international boundaries. This "unlock" was equally revolutionary in its impact, fundamentally changing how the world responds to health threats and coordinates health improvement efforts on a global scale.

A New Model for Global Health Coordination

Parallel to the development of the domestic healthcare market in the US, the post-World War II period saw the creation of new international organizations designed to address global challenges with coordinated action. The most significant of these for public health was the World Health Organization (WHO), whose constitution came into force in April 1948. The establishment of the WHO represented a fundamental shift in how the international community approached health challenges. Unlike previous international health efforts, which had been primarily focused on bilateral arrangements, the WHO was designed to coordinate global health efforts through a centralized organizational structure. The first World Health Assembly, held in 1948, included representatives from 53 member states. This assembly established the precedent for global decision-making on health issues and created the institutional framework that would enable coordinated international health initiatives. The timing of WHO's establishment, just as global communications technology was beginning to develop, was crucial for the organization's eventual success in coordinating worldwide health efforts.

Smallpox Eradication

The most compelling example of the

transformative impact of global communications on public health is the World Health Organization's Smallpox Eradication Program. This initiative represented the first successful global eradication of a human disease, demonstrating how improved communications technology enabled unprecedented coordination of health activities across the world. An expansive, worldwide smallpox eradication program was announced by the World Health Assembly in 1958. The program was formally put forth by the Soviet Union's representative and passed by a majority vote by member states, demonstrating the shared global commitment to this ambitious undertaking.

The organizational structure of the smallpox eradication program was specifically designed to enable centralized coordination while allowing for regional and national adaptation. The World Health Organization Headquarters in Geneva worked alongside regional offices to engage national governments and citizens to ensure success. This multi-level coordination system was only possible due to the global communications infrastructure built at the beginning of the US I global world order.

The smallpox eradication program employed several coordination mechanisms that would have been impossible without advanced communications technology. These included:

- **Global Surveillance Systems**: The program required rapid reporting of smallpox cases from remote areas around the world to central coordination centers. This surveillance system needed to operate in real-time to enable quick response to outbreaks and to track the progress of eradication efforts.
- **Standardized Response Protocols**: The same eradication methods and strategies were repeated in very different countries around the globe. This standardization required continuous communication between field operations and central coordination centers to ensure

consistency and effectiveness.

- **Resource Coordination**: The program involved the coordinated deployment of vaccines, personnel, and other resources across multiple countries and continents. This coordination required sophisticated logistics and communication systems to ensure that resources were available where and when they were needed.
- **Progress Monitoring**: Continuous assessment of program effectiveness across regions required regular communication of detailed epidemiological data from field operations to central analysis centers. This monitoring was essential for making strategic adjustments to the program and for maintaining international support and funding.

The success of the smallpox eradication program was unprecedented in the history of public health. Smallpox was officially declared eradicated in

1980, making it the first disease to have been successfully fought on a global scale. This was accomplished through the collaboration of countries around the world and represented a new model for addressing global health challenges. The smallpox program's success demonstrated the potential for centralized global health coordination when supported by adequate communications technology. The ability to coordinate activities across continents, share information in real-time, and maintain consistent strategies across diverse cultural and political contexts proved that global health challenges could be addressed through coordinated international action.

Institutionalization of Global Health Coordination

The success of early global health coordination efforts led to the institutionalization of centralized coordination as a standard approach to addressing global health challenges. Organizations like WHO expanded coordination capabilities and developed more sophisticated systems for managing global health initiatives. This institutionalization was supported by continued improvements in communications technology, which made coordination activities more efficient and effective over time. The integration of communications technology into the standard operating procedures of global health organizations became a defining characteristic of modern global health systems.

The global disease surveillance and communication systems developed to combat smallpox were applied to other global health initiatives, including efforts to control malaria, tuberculosis, and other infectious diseases. These programs all relied on the same basic coordination structure: centralized planning and oversight combined with regional and national implementation, all connected through sophisticated communications systems. The success of these coordination mechanisms led to their adoption beyond infectious disease control. Global health initiatives addressing maternal and child health, nutrition, and other health issues began to employ similar approaches, demonstrating the broad applicability of centralized coordination supported by global communications. This real-time capability was particularly important for surveillance and monitoring activities, which required rapid reporting of health data from field locations to central analysis centers. The speed of satellite communications made it possible to detect and respond to health threats much more quickly than had been possible with previous technology.

Long-term Impact

Both the rise of for-profit healthcare businesses and the development of global public health organizations unlocked lasting positive impacts on the healthcare system. These impacts extended far beyond specific programs like smallpox eradication and influenced how the overall healthcare system operated.

The for-profit healthcare business model fundamentally transformed the US healthcare market from fragmented and underfunded local hospitals into efficient, technology-enabled, integrated health systems. This wasn't just a change in ownership structure - it was a complete redesign of how healthcare would work. Given the extent of the positive impacts, we discuss them across four themes:

1. Unlocking Capital to Build Modern Health Systems
2. Improved Organizational Design
3. Driving Innovation Adoption
4. Government Collaboration and Partnership

Theme #1: Unlocking Capital to Build Modern Health Systems

One of the most significant impacts of the burgeoning for-profit healthcare industry was its revolutionary ability to mobilize capital for healthcare infrastructure. Unlike traditional non-profit hospitals that relied on donations and government funding, for-profit health systems could access vastly more capital through equity and debt markets. This influx of capital enabled large-scale technological advancement and standardization across networks, as these chains were often the earliest adopters of new medical technologies, integrating them systematically into their facilities. For instance, HCA heavily invested in comprehensive medical data systems accessible at both hospitals and physicians' offices, creating integrated information networks that enhanced care coordination and business operations. This competitive pressure spurred all hospitals, regardless of their ownership structure, to modernize their facilities and improve services, fostering an environment of continuous improvement across the entire industry.

The synergistic effects of the two unlocks created efficiency gains and cost optimization opportunities that neither could have achieved alone. For-profit organizations' capital investment spurred market competition, pushing all providers to find efficiency improvements in healthcare delivery. Simultaneously, coordination mechanisms developed for global public health were adapted to strengthen communication between the corporate offices and the many hospitals, clinics, and ambulatory centers distributed across the US. Competitive pressures introduced by for-profit providers compelled all healthcare organizations to enhance efficiency and service quality. While new communication systems facilitated the standardization and sharing of evidence-based practices across extensive healthcare delivery networks, improving overall care.

Theme #2: Improved Organizational Design

Another crucial strategic innovation developed by for-profit chains was the creation of mechanisms to align physician interests with hospital operations. Traditional nonprofit hospitals often struggled with the fact that physicians, who controlled patient admissions and treatment decisions, were not employees of the hospital and therefore had limited financial incentives to consider hospital efficiency or profit margins. For-profit health systems addressed this challenge through various physician alignment strategies. HCA, for example, developed multiple strategies to include local physicians in profit-sharing and equity ownership structures. They were not the only for-profit to work to align incentives to drive efficiency - most, if not all, for-profit systems pursued similar strategies.

Depending on one's perspective, for-profit organizations led the way (or pushed the boundary) in aligning financial interests with doctors. These integration strategies were carefully designed to comply with anti-kickback laws and ethical guidelines prohibiting direct payments for patient referrals. However, the regulations are complex and nuanced, and the incentive programs are highly structured. This resulted in fines to HCA and others over the many decades of the industry's growth and development. However, there is no question that the entry of for-profit organizations into the health delivery market caused the industry to become much more aligned around the combination of both patient care and financial strength.

For-profit healthcare systems also pioneered the integration of multiple service offerings, extending operations beyond traditional inpatient services to include a full continuum of healthcare services. This vertical integration approach represented a fundamental shift from the fragmented healthcare delivery that had characterized the pre-war period. Companies like HCA created integrated networks that included not only hospitals but also ambulatory surgical centers, diagnostic facilities, home care affiliates, and rehabilitation facilities. This integration enabled coordination of care across different settings and service types, improving both the quality and efficiency of healthcare delivery. The integration strategies developed by for-profit chains influenced the broader healthcare system, leading to increased emphasis on coordinated care delivery and the development of integrated delivery systems across all types of healthcare providers.

At the same time, improvements in global communication networks enabled data sharing and the standardization of public health approaches across different regions. This enabled the development of evidence-based practices that could be applied consistently across diverse settings, facilitated the sharing of expertise and resources among countries, and created opportunities for comparative evaluation of diverse approaches to similar health challenges. However, it has also raised ongoing questions about the appropriateness of standardized approaches in diverse cultural, economic, and political contexts. The tension between standardization and local adaptation remains a central challenge today. The balance between achieving the benefits of standardization and maintaining the flexibility necessary for local adaptation continues to be an area of focus.

These two core organizational changes, incentive alignment and integrated networks, were initially combined in various ways by for-profit organizations and subsequently adopted by nonprofit health systems. Over time, this led to the development of new organizational models that integrated market-based and coordination-based approaches to match the needs of the health system and the community. These hybrid organizational models became characteristic of modern healthcare systems and represented a significant innovation in organizational design.

Theme #3: Driving Innovation Adoption

The for-profit, healthcare service delivery models and coordinated global public health planning created accelerated innovation cycles and systematic problem-solving capabilities. In healthcare, much of this innovation focused on process improvements and regulatory innovation. For-profit health systems were early adopters of new processes designed to more effectively and efficiently care for patients. Unlike product innovations, these changes can be challenging to observe from the outside. This is because innovation often lies in how patients are moved through the healthcare system, eliminating wait-states or inefficient steps from the overall process. Another type of innovation that drove the healthcare market is regulatory innovation.

As mentioned previously, the primary reimbursement model used by the US government for Medicare was a cost-plus model during the 1960s and 1970s. However, as the industry grew in size, the significant expenditure drew attention, and politicians began seeking a more effective payment method. In 1982, Medicare reimbursement was changed to payment based on a fixed amount for each healthcare procedure. Of course, the implementation of a fixed price for healthcare is inherently complicated by the fact that each patient is unique and presents distinct health concerns. Proper healthcare treatment requires a physician to provide customized care to each patient. US regulators attempted to solve this using a system based on Diagnosis-Related Groups (DRGs). The DRG system established a patient classification scheme providing a means of defining and standardizing the type of patients a hospital treats.

The new system changed Medicare reimbursement from paying the cost plus a margin percentage to instead reimbursing providers with a fixed payment amount based on the patient's diagnosis. This system shifted the financial risk to healthcare systems. If the healthcare organizations spend more on delivering the service than the fixed DRG payment, they would lose money. Yet it also drove a focus on efficiency. If a healthcare provider could treat patients for less expense than the DRG fixed reimbursement, they could keep the difference as profit. This regulatory change caused a "Cambrian explosion" in the number and diversity of for-profit healthcare businesses. Jack Massey, while still on the Board of Directors of HCA, formed the venture capital firm Massey Burch & Company to invest in high-growth healthcare startups in the Nashville area. One of the venture investments was Surgical Care Affiliates (SCA). This company was established to provide a specific set of surgical procedures on an outpatient basis. Two experienced Nashville healthcare executives, Joel Gordon and Andrew "Woody" Miller, created SCA in 1982 with financial backing from Massey Burch. The company excels by providing a superior patient experience, and by focusing on a limited set of procedures, they have been able to generate substantial profits by significantly reducing their costs below DRG reimbursement rates. SCA went public in an IPO only two years later, in 1984, and was eventually sold in 1996 to HealthSouth for $1.1 billion.

Market mechanisms, spurred by the for-profit competition, provided incentives for the adoption of innovation. For-profit healthcare enterprises were early adopters of process and regulatory innovations, leveraging these advantages to gain a competitive edge and grow rapidly. The nonprofit healthcare systems worked to keep up, resulting in the healthcare industry becoming more efficient and far larger during this period. The combination of innovation incentives and rapid diffusion mechanisms created a powerful engine for the growth of the healthcare industry, accelerating the pace of innovation.

Theme #4: Government Collaboration and Partnership

The development of global communications technology enabled a fundamental shift in public health to truly multilateral, global coordination mechanisms.
This shift created opportunities for addressing health

challenges that transcended national boundaries and required coordinated responses across multiple countries simultaneously. The success of the smallpox eradication program demonstrated that global health challenges could be addressed through coordinated international action when supported by an adequate communications infrastructure.

Collaboration and partnerships between all healthcare providers, whether for-profit or non-profit, and governments were critically valuable. The key to success was to establish trust between the community and the health system delivering care. Difficult healthcare allocation decisions often need to be made, but they are best navigated through transparent communication and shared values. To this end, as the for-profit model developed, challenges and debates arose over what is fair and who should pay for care. This requires clear policy and regulatory actions or collaborations aimed at addressing concerns about access, quality, and market competition. These included regulations governing hospital conversions from non-profit to for-profit status, requirements for community benefit programs, and various quality measurement and reporting requirements. This regulatory framework eventually developed into a critical part of the overall healthcare policy landscape, influencing both healthcare and public health, regardless of their ownership structure.

The interaction between market-based healthcare delivery and coordinated global public health planning created accelerated innovation cycles, enhancing the pace of healthcare advancement. Market mechanisms provided incentives for innovation, while global coordination mechanisms enabled rapid diffusion and testing of innovations across diverse contexts. For-profit healthcare enterprises were motivated to develop innovative approaches to healthcare delivery to maintain a competitive advantage. The global communications infrastructure enabled these innovations to be shared rapidly with other providers worldwide, creating larger markets for innovations and providing feedback that could be used to refine and improve them.

Elevate Health Vision for 2050:

The adoption of technical and process innovations by for-profit healthcare businesses during the last significant step forward in human health, 1945-1970, led to the fastest positive changes in global human health and wellness. We understand that they were able to build alongside the positive momentum of the emergence of a single globally optimized world order (US I) to improve health metrics worldwide. The Elevate Health 2050 community is dedicated to studying how these changes came about and aspires to help shape the next such emergence. In 2050, during the next "High Turning," no matter who emerges from the chaos and fighting expected in the Crisis, the Elevate Health 2050 community will be there.

Many members of the EH community are concerned about health issues of life and death every day. Elevate Health applauds these dedicated health caregivers. However, our focus is longer dated. We aim to install value-based health systems in every significant new community or healthcare-affiliated group over the next 25 years. These communities can use any or all parts of the Elevate Health model. As in open-source software, future Elevate Health adopters may also build new features on top of the core EH Market Attributes. Each community may have very different religious, cultural, or political belief systems. This is expected. The point is to elevate health above these petty squabbles. This book aspires to grow into an instruction manual of sorts.

Consider a future President of the US in the year 2050. She is a millennial woman. The US has regained its position as the global leader in AI, Web3, and Biotech innovations, effectively controlling over 50% of the health and care sector. This is achieved through an independent third party responsible for the Health and well-being of the population, utilizing numerous metrics as reasonable. This president turns to the cameras and directly calls for help in delivering the best possible healthcare to the people. Money is no object. The government creates USD to pay. Yet, behavior change is only partially susceptible to financial incentives. This book, Elevate Health 2050, is intended to serve as a "paint-by-numbers" manual for the future leader of the free world. This period will require a thorough understanding of the technological waves of AI, Web 3, and Biotech. They also need to learn from the past to shape the next step in societal evolution.

Lessons from the Last Cycle

The innovations examined in this chapter offer important

lessons for the Elevate Health community as it addresses future health challenges. Market forces drive innovation and growth, but they are insufficient for ensuring equitable access. Government and regulatory policy must establish societal norms such as equal access to healthcare. We observe that following World War II, the US achieved this combination of market forces with policy regulation. This occurred naturally and without any grand design or coordinated effort. Partially, this was a natural outgrowth of American idealism and President Johnson's pursuit of the Great Society. Still, it also emerged through a series of unintended consequences and fortunate turns of history. As we begin to apply the lessons of the last cycle to build the Elevate Health Community, we cannot rely on an as-yet unknown future world power to follow this idealistic and constructive path. Nor are we comfortable leaving our future healthcare markets to favorable happenstance.

Addressing future global health challenges such as chronic disease management, genetic treatments, and end-of-life care will be complex as they will be both intensely personal and critically important to most. We anticipate that challenges will require a similar balance of methods to what we saw in the last cycle. Some mechanisms will be needed to improve and expand healthcare services, while others will need to ensure equity and fairness for all. Elevate Health must develop means to harness the power of the coming three waves of technical innovation through market and profit-motive forces. Yet we also must develop guidelines and regulations to establish a new set of societal norms and then enforce these norms through policy and compliance.

During the last cycle, the most successful approaches combined market pressures with public coordination, private innovation with standardized implementation, and local delivery with global coordination. This finding has important implications for future healthcare markets. The most effective healthcare systems for our shared future will come from the integration of multiple approaches aligned and optimized to improve health outcomes and quality of life for all. Historical experience suggests that the most effective strategies to address the coming healthcare challenges will be those that successfully integrate multiple mechanisms and capabilities, rather than relying on any single approach.

The lessons learned from post-war innovations serve as valuable guides as we turn our attention to addressing future healthcare challenges.

Chapter 4: Shared Values and Beliefs

Remain true to your values. If you don't stand for something, you'll fall for anything.

– Frank Sonnenberg

In the last chapter, we discussed the two health unlocks of the last cycle. This evaluation uncovered the insight that effective future health markets will need to integrate mechanisms, incentives, and regulations to balance the drive for innovation and growth with equity and fairness. As we apply these lessons to create the Elevate Health Community, we must do so without relying on any single government or regulatory body. This is the opportunity and challenge of launching the Elevate Health effort before the next crisis and subsequent high period.

In the last cycle, the crisis was the "one-two punch" of the Great Depression, combined with the violence and fear of a world war initiated by Germany and Japan. In Neil Howe's cycle, it is this global crisis that brings all of society together against a common enemy. The shared and intensely emotional experience focuses our collective effort during the crisis and enables the high period thereafter. Almost no one alive today experienced the last crisis. If we imagine an 18-year-old entering the military in 1945, this person would be 98 years old today. Very few WWII veterans are still alive today. The Boomer generation is, of course, named for the "baby boom" that occurred following the war. Therefore, as Howe describes, we now have four generations, including Boomers, X-Gen, Millennials, and Gen Z, that have never experienced a true global crisis.

We observe the rise of extremist and populist movements in the US and around the world. These are concerning trends; however, we have not yet escalated into a full-blown crisis. The challenge of launching Elevate Health in the run-up to the future crisis is that, by definition, our various cultural, political, and religious affiliations seem essential, making it difficult or impossible to reach a shared consensus. Elevate Health is NOT attempting to build a shared society analogous to President Johnson's attempt at creating the Great Society. Nor do we expect to establish a shared consensus on culturally, politically, and religiously charged health issues such as genetic modification and the abortion debate. We believe this to be impossible until after the upcoming crisis. Furthermore, we see an opportunity to foster multiple Elevate Health-affiliated groups that agree on most health issues but disagree on a relatively few based on cultural, political, or religious beliefs.

We choose to focus on what we share in common, not our few differences. Through this focus on shared values and beliefs, we seek to pull or "elevate" health issues above these cultural, political, and religious differences. The hope is that before the crisis, many of the fractured societal groups will adopt the Elevate Health shared values and foundational beliefs. Not because there is any alignment or agreement on how we govern ourselves. Instead, the Elevate Health Community aims to educate and inform its members about how these values and beliefs enhance health and wellness, regardless of one's other cultural, political, and religious beliefs.

We include the year 2050 in the book's title to remind ourselves of the Elevate Health Community's long-term perspective on healthcare policy development. The transformative changes examined in this research took decades to fully develop.. This is one of the reasons we have elected to focus on the health markets of 2050. Significant and structural changes can only be accomplished over long time horizons. However, the opportunity is immense with the health and wellness of 5 billion people and $5 trillion in annual global market revenues at stake.

As we prepare to elevate health and fully capitalize on the next window of opportunity, the lessons from the last cycle suggest that transformative health system change requires the alignment of several enabling conditions, including supportive policy frameworks, technological capabilities, and institutional innovations. In the second half of the book, we will focus on defining and creating these enabling conditions rather than leaving our shared health future to chance. In chapter 2, we introduced the concept of a "societal medium." This medium is characterized by active human agency, collective decision-making, and emergent behaviors that continuously reshape its properties. We call it a medium because of how it shapes, channels, and constrains the innovation waves. In this chapter, we address what it means to start a new global health market and then describe the two primary components of this societal medium: shared values and foundational beliefs. We end the chapter by introducing three representatives to help us gain a perspective of how this new healthcare experience feels to Elevate Health Community members.

Bootstrapping a new Healthcare Market

Elevate Health 2050 is attempting to bootstrap a new global health market from scratch. We believe that as the innovation waves of AI, Web3, and BioTech begin to arrive, it will be possible for a relatively small community to successfully launch an entirely new market.

The Elevate Health 2050 Vision:

1. Elevate health above politics
2. Align around shared health values and beliefs
3. Start by ending heart disease

It has not previously been possible to bootstrap an entirely new market. Yet the capabilities enabled by AI and Web3 technology are accelerating quickly. Small teams of builders have never been so powerful. We are not planning for some distant future. Instead, we assert that we can start now, today. Yes, it will take time, and incumbents will resist. But we must begin and learn as much as possible as quickly as possible.

If Neil Howe and Ray Dalio are correct, our society will hit a crisis period at some point in the next 5-15 years. We cannot predict how this crisis will emerge. It could take many forms, such as a financial crisis, civil unrest, international conflict, or a full-scale war. However, we believe that our best chance to "elevate health" above politics is to establish a set of shared values and beliefs

before the crisis arrives. This window of opportunity only occurs once every four generations. Our community aims to maximize this opportunity to elevate health, moving it away from dependency and reliance on the State or Employer. Our first shared value is that Health is a Human Right. We refuse to risk giving up our health and personal sovereignty to petty political or religious differences. In this pursuit, we begin developing the Elevate Health market today, with full implementation planned for 2050. We selected this year because our society will (we hope) have survived the coming global crisis and will be entering the new High period.

Bootstrapping

Bootstrapping is a term typically used in the context of entrepreneurship. It refers to the process of starting and growing a business with minimal external funding or capital. Essentially, it means utilizing your own resources, including personal savings, sweat equity, and revenue generated by the business, to fund operations and drive growth. Entrepreneurs typically choose to bootstrap a new business in order to maintain control and not be forced to raise capital from investors. While this is a choice for startups, we believe it is a requirement for the successful development of an independent health market. This is the only path that creates a self-sufficient market with no investors and no outside influencers.

As we start to bootstrap the Elevate Health Market for 2050, there are several characteristics of bootstrapped companies that we should consider and adapt to our purposes:

- **Self-reliance:** Bootstrapped companies rely on internal financial resources to launch and grow. Therefore, Elevate Health will need to develop methods to finance the infrastructure and support systems necessary for the market to serve its participants effectively.
- **Frugality:** Bootstrapped companies emphasize minimizing costs and maximizing efficiency. This follows naturally from the self-reliance; Elevate Health will need to be frugal and highly efficient.
- **Organic growth:** Growth at bootstrapped companies is fueled by internal resources and reinvestment of profits, rather than external investments. Elevate Health must also develop organic and self-financing methods to grow members and market reach. This may lead to a slow rate of growth, but we prefer slow and steady growth to protect our community's independence.

Open-source Community Model

Elevate Health 2050 will utilize the open-source community model as a framework to inform the assembly of our community. These communities share much in common with our vision. They are bootstrapped, built by a group of passionate community members, and allow anyone to join and use the community resources. Open-source projects often begin with a small group of passionate individuals who contribute their time and skills voluntarily. They typically lack significant financial resources or institutional backing. Over time, the open-source community grows organically as more contributors and users become involved, developing software, documentation, and support. This growth is driven by shared enthusiasm and collaboration, not external investment. The community collectively owns and maintains the project, with no single entity controlling its direction. This decentralized approach aligns with the bootstrapping ethos of self-reliance and shared responsibility.

WordPress Community Illustration:

From its earliest days, WordPress was more than just software—it was a community united by shared values and ideals. The early WordPress community was small but passionate. Contributors gathered on mailing lists and topic channels, sharing code, ideas, and a vision for making web publishing accessible to everyone. Unlike many open-source projects that focused primarily on technical excellence, WordPress, from the beginning, prioritized user experience and ease of use. This focus was sometimes controversial among developers who preferred more technically sophisticated solutions, but it proved to be one of WordPress's most significant strategic advantages.

The early WordPress community developed practices that would become templates for open-source collaboration at scale. Code contributions were welcomed from anyone, but they underwent rigorous review processes that maintained quality standards. Documentation was treated as equally valuable to code, recognizing that software is only as good as people's ability to use it effectively. The community began developing the inclusive culture that would later enable WordPress to build one of the most diverse contributor bases in open-source software. Perhaps most importantly, the early community established patterns of decision-making that balanced technical expertise with user needs. While technical contributors had significant influence over implementation details, major decisions about WordPress's direction were made with careful consideration of how they would affect the broader user community. This user-centric approach would prove crucial as WordPress evolved from a blogging platform to a comprehensive content management system.

Perhaps most significantly, this period saw the emergence of WordCamp, the community conference system that would become a cornerstone of the WordPress community. The first WordCamp, held in San Francisco in 2006, brought together fewer than 500 people. However, it established a template for community events that would eventually span the globe, providing regular opportunities for in-person collaboration and relationship-building that strengthened the bonds of the distributed WordPress community.

As WordPress's global community grew, it was primarily supported by the expansion of the WordCamp conference system. From a single annual event, WordCamps grew to dozens of conferences held around the world, each organized by local communities but following consistent global standards. This approach enabled community building at scale while respecting local cultural differences and needs. The WordCamp model demonstrated innovative thinking about how to scale community events without compromising their personal and collaborative character. Rather than creating a centralized conference organization, the WordPress community developed guidelines and support systems that enabled local organizers to create events tailored to their specific communities, while maintaining the values and quality standards that define the WordPress experience.

Today, WordPress has a significant global impact. The platform powers over 40% of all websites, supports more than 2 million contributors, and generates an estimated annual economic impact of over $600 billion. WordPress's approach to community building demonstrates a sophisticated understanding of how to maintain shared values and collaborative practices across diverse cultural and geographic contexts. The community has successfully scaled from a small group of like-minded individuals to a global network of millions while preserving the collaborative spirit and inclusive values that defined its early culture. As Elevate Health begins to build our community, there is much to take from the WordPress example.

Align Around Shared Health Values:

As we navigate uncertain times and face potential crises, we call on all individuals, communities, and nations to unite around a shared vision for healthcare. We believe that health is a fundamental human right, and we must work together to create a healthcare market that is sustainable, equitable, and innovative.

Values align the Elevate Health community members in bootstrapping and building our health markets independent of specific strategies and tactics. This creative tension is critically important to make clear to all members and potential members. Elevate Health is an open community. This means that anyone and everyone is welcome to join and become a member. The only requirement is that all members must ascribe to our shared health values and foundational beliefs. However, when it comes to implementation details, including how to allocate healthcare resources, how to fund healthcare services, which specific treatments should be provided to population groups, and a myriad of other operational details, Elevate Health is open-minded and willing to test any ideas.

We expect broad debate and uncertainty over issues related to how best to implement, allocate, and regulate health. Yet, if we can agree on shared values, we believe our community will improve human health more rapidly and fairly in the next 25 years.

Our Shared Values:

1. **Health is a Human Right:** Everyone deserves access to quality healthcare, regardless of their background or circumstances.
2. **Sustainable Funding and Allocation:** We must fund our healthcare system for the long term, ensuring equitable access for current and future generations.
3. **Aligned Incentives and Innovation:** We must foster collaboration and innovation to optimize resources and deliver the best possible care.

We owe it to our children and grandchildren to build a healthier world.

Beliefs Shape the Market:

Aligning efforts around core values helps to connect and align our community, but it isn't enough. Elevate Health also holds Foundational Beliefs to help shape the market in a positive direction and drive positive change. This approach will foster trust between patients and healthcare providers, creating a foundation for a more collaborative and effective healthcare system. Ultimately, this will create a health market in 2050 that prioritizes patient needs and ethical, sustainable practices.

Elevate Health 2050 Foundational Beliefs:

1. **High and Low Margin Business Categories:** The For-Profit vs. Non-Profit dichotomy is a false choice. It implies that some organizations are working to "make money," and others are "helping people." This is inaccurate and unfair to both sides. We believe markets will evolve over the next 25 years to adopt one of two organizational types in the Elevate Health Market of 2050: High-Margin and Low-Margin.
2. **Radical Market Transparency and Personal Data Sovereignty:** Healthcare debates are challenging, specifically due to the emotional intensity and deeply held beliefs. Too often, these differences cause us to focus too much

attention and energy on our points of contention, rather than on our shared values. The unprecedented capabilities of the Intelligence Age will necessitate the exploration of new governance and resource allocation models. This adds to the complexity and increases the stakes. We believe the best method for navigating these emotionally charged and intensely personal topics is through Radical Market Transparency, combined with Personal Data Sovereignty.

3. **Race to the Top for Health:** Elevate Health aims to apply the "Race to the Top" framework, developed by Anthropic, to promote collaboration, competition, and transparency within the health market. By encouraging the sharing of knowledge and best practices, we accelerate the development of innovative solutions, leading to earlier diagnoses, more accurate assessments, and optimized treatments. This collaborative environment will also help reduce health disparities by mitigating biases in healthcare algorithms and ensuring equitable access to care for all populations.

Belief #1: Upgrading outdated For-profit / Non-profit Categories

The for-profit model in healthcare during the last cycle, while controversial, catalyzed unprecedented innovation, access, and financial sustainability, but also introduced ethical dilemmas and inequities. While the for-profit model has led to significant benefits in healthcare, it will need to be either constrained or aligned to meet the new demands of fairness held by the Millennial and Gen Z generations. We believe in the power of aligned incentives to drive individuals and organizations toward positive behaviors and outcomes.

While a shared set of values will be helpful, it will not be sufficient. Profit motives must be aligned with non-profit missions by creating a framework in which for-profit companies actively contribute to non-profits' public health missions while benefiting one another in a win-win scenario. Simply incentives reduce the chance of unintended consequences, but simple does not imply easy. It is challenging to design a simple yet effective set of incentives. We suggest the creation of a community designed to create a robust ecosystem where for-profit and non-profit entities are aligned, fostering collaboration to address pressing public health and personal healthcare challenges. If incentives can be designed properly, this community can spur innovation, leverage diverse resources, and maximize impact for all.

By clearly establishing alignment between for-profit and non-profit healthcare models, we can launch a positive flywheel of health and healthcare, driving improvements in public health (non-profit models) and personal healthcare (for-profit and non-profit models).

High-margin and low-margin organizations:
The Elevate Health Community believes we must upgrade the outdated labels of "For-profit" and "Non-profit" organizations to the clearer and accurate categories of "High-Margin" and "Low-Margin" organizations. While the for-profit model has led to significant benefits to healthcare, it will need to be either constrained or aligned to meet the new demands of fairness held by the Millennial and younger generations as we enter the Intelligence Age. The EH Community believes in the power of aligned incentives to drive individuals and organizations toward positive behaviors and outcomes. Our shared values will be helpful, but ultimately insufficient to engender trust and ensure alignment. Healthcare is emotionally charged and intensely personal. Public opinion has been trending negatively against Private Equity, PBMs, and large for-profit health insurers. This culminated with the murder of Brian Thompson, CEO of United Healthcare in December 2024. Our community needs to trust that we understand the distinctions between for-profit and non-profit structures, ensuring alignment that allows for-profit

businesses to contribute positively to our community's values and goals.

The For-Profit vs. Non-Profit dichotomy is a false choice. It implies that some organizations are working to “make money,” and others are “helping people.” This is inaccurate and unfair to both sides. By definition, all members of EH 2050 are working to Elevate Health and help people. Additionally, all organizations must generate sufficient revenue and a gross margin to cover the necessary overhead, including personnel, equipment, and facilities. Of course, some organizations and some products or business models are naturally more profitable than others. However, no responsible organization and leadership team would approve a budget that completely “runs out of money” precisely at the end of the year. All organizations must generate revenue to finance operations and create savings or profits, ensuring that the people, equipment, and buildings can be supported and maintained. We can do better.

All Elevate Health organizations should be aligned using a framework in which highly profitable companies contribute innovation and new products, while low-margin organizations, whether for-profit or non-profit under US tax law, contribute by delivering public health and wellness products and services to members. Clear, simple, and aligned incentives reduce the chance of unintended consequences and mistrust. We suggest the Elevate Health community proactively design a transparent & aligned market where for-profit and non-profit evolve over the next 25 years to adopt one of two organizational types in the Elevate Health Market of 2050: High-Margin and Low-Margin.

- High-Margin: The first category of organizations in the EH 2050 community is the High-Margin category. This is an intentionally broad definition because, as we build the entire healthcare market infrastructure over the next 25 years, we expect to need many doctors and nurses, as well as software developers, health coaches, capital allocators, venture capitalists, bankers, lawyers, and scientists, to name a few. High-Margin organizations are innovative and often capture high gross margins. There are no restrictions on High-Margin organizations. However, as a way to contribute to the overall Elevate Health 2050 vision, they are required to contribute 10% of their revenues in the form of either free services or educational content. We want our partners to actively build an educational marketing and customer conversion system. The more High-Margin organizations earn through Elevate Health markets, the closer we get to our goal of $5 trillion total market size in 2050, and the more these organizations invest in the community through the 10% requirement.

- Low-Margin: Low-Margin organizations exist to deliver established but undifferentiated public health, wellness, diagnostic, and preventive services, while also conducting medical procedures. The Low-Margin organization type is required to maintain gross margins of under 15%, averaged across all its products and weighted by revenue size. Often, former Non-Profit organizations will have systems, products, and services suited to this category of Elevate Health. That is great, we want to collaborate to address pressing public health and personal healthcare challenges.

Importantly, both categories of Elevate Health organizations will access capital markets. High-Margin organizations fit well with VC, PE, and public stock markets. At the same time, Low-Margin organizations will be more suited to debt and bond markets. Both types of organizations will benefit from the collective buying power of the community. With this clear and straightforward incentive structure, both kinds of organizations contribute to strengthening the community.

High-margin organizations are well-suited to driving new and innovative methods for diagnosing, treating, and managing healthcare issues. They attract talent and capital to the healthcare industry by providing the opportunity for significant profit for shareholders and net worth appreciation for individuals. However, public health and routine implementation of established healthcare practices typically produce the most benefits to health and wellness outcomes when they are offered at a low cost to everyone. These activities are best suited for low-margin organizations.

By clearly establishing alignment between Low-Margin and High-Margin healthcare models, we can launch a positive flywheel of health and healthcare, driving improvements in public health and wellness (primarily non-profit models) and advanced, specialized, and innovative healthcare procedures (typically for-profit models).

Incentive Structures

Our framing of organizational types within the Elevate Health community is foundational, as it enables us to develop an aligned incentive structure tailored to each group. The clarity and freedom provided by such a transparent shared understanding across all members of the community will be empowering to everyone.

High-Margin Incentive Structure

High-Margin organizations are welcome in the Elevate Health community as long as they

1. Ascribe to our community values and
2. Contribution Commitment: Companies must commit to donating:

    - 10% of the revenue earned from the Elevate Health community must be donated as resources (in-kind services, research, cash, etc.) to support public health initiatives.

Benefits of Participating for High-Margin Companies:

- Patient/Customer Referrals: We introduce potential customers to the free public health utility and design an upgrade pathway for those who can afford to pay.
- Social Impact Branding: Association with the public health utility enhances their brand image and demonstrates their commitment to social responsibility.
- Access to Network & Resources: Gain access to the EH Community's network of experts, researchers, patients, and community partners.
- Collaboration Opportunities: Engage in collaborative projects and initiatives that align with your expertise and interests.

<u>Low-Margin Incentive Structure</u>

Low-Margin organizations are welcome in the Elevate Health community as long as they

1. Ascribe to our values and
2. Provide health and wellness services with gross margins of less than 15% on revenue earned from the EH community. This limitation of non-profit gross margins is designed to focus resources on

areas of public health and routine implementation of established healthcare practices. The 15% is taken from the Medical Loss Ratio embedded in the ACA for insurers.

Benefits of Participating for Low-Margin Organizations:

- Sustainable Free Public Health Utilities: Secure diversified and ongoing programs of all types to bring health to all humans, no matter their wealth and status.
- Expertise & Resources: Access valuable expertise, resources, and innovative solutions from the private sector. Some companies may be willing to donate services such as training, coaching, teaching, providing care, advising others, etc.
- Collaboration & Innovation: Foster partnerships that can accelerate progress and lead to new solutions for public health challenges. Offer research grants to both nonprofits and for-profit organizations that join the community.
- Increased Visibility: Expand the reach and impact of the Low-Margin's mission through collaborative marketing and outreach efforts.

This belief contributes to Elevate Health's sustainability and self-reliance: As we learned through the WordPress example, bootstrapped and open-source communities must rely on internally generated financial resources to launch and grow. By developing the High-Margin and

Low-Margin organizational categories, Elevate Health inherently sets up the process by which our community finances the establishment of infrastructure and support systems necessary for the market to effectively serve its participants. High-margin organizations must contribute 10% of revenues generated from the Elevate Health Market back into improving it for all. Low-margin organizations provide a means to allow basic services that Elevate Health calls "utilities" to members in a sustainable manner.

Why 10% Community Investment

It is essential to explain why we believe that 10% is the right level of required community investment by high-profit Margin organizations. In the long term, the Elevate Health markets will invest 10% into public health and primary care delivered through the AI Coach interface and all of the free and inexpensive health and wellness services available on the Markets. When we consider the IP policy changes and the Race to the Top culture, Elevate Health expects to increase the free value to all members each year. In addition, the US health industry spends about 5% on primary care today and some amount, albeit not enough, on publc health. Doubling this level to 10% seems to be a valuable signal that primary care and public health is essential to overall health and wellness. Yet we also expect to deliver the care with far better efficiency. This will allow Elevate Health to deliver more than double the health and wellness value to members. From the perspective of high-profit organizations, the 10% is reflective of religious tithe giving and can be an ongoing aspect of a healthy organization.

Belief #2: Radical Market Transparency and Personal Data Sovereignty

Healthcare debates are challenging, specifically due to the emotional intensity and deeply held beliefs. Differing worldviews, shaped by religious beliefs, social norms, and political ideologies, are natural; however, these differences often cause us to focus too much attention and energy on our points of contention, rather than our shared values. Add to this the financial complexities of balancing cost, access, and quality, along with the overwhelming deluge of misinformation, and it becomes clear why finding common ground in health becomes so difficult. We are at a moment in time where we see the fractioning of social and political groups, and a disconnect between the rich and the poor. These forces challenge existing norms in healthcare and various aspects of our lives.

The unprecedented capabilities of these three waves of innovation in AI, Web3, and Biotech will necessitate the exploration of new governance and resource allocation models. This adds to the complexity and increases the stakes. We will need to devise new regulatory frameworks, ethical guidelines, and resource allocation strategies to ensure these three powerful innovations are used responsibly and equitably in healthcare. Yet the very purpose of the Elevate Health 2050 community is to elevate health, not to antagonize all sides. We aim to navigate these emotionally charged and intensely personal topics with our 2nd Foundational Belief of Radical Transparency combined with Personal Data Privacy.

Broken Status Quo

The current landscape of health data management is fraught with challenges and vulnerabilities, mainly stemming from its centralized nature. Hospitals, insurance companies, and electronic health record (EHR) providers hold vast amounts of sensitive patient data, making them prime targets for cyberattacks, such as ransomware and data breaches. This centralization creates single points of failure, where a breach in one system can compromise millions of records. Beyond security risks, the lack of interoperability across these fragmented systems leads to incomplete patient records and significant inefficiencies in care delivery. Perhaps most concerning is the limited patient control; individuals often have little to no direct say in who accesses, uses, or shares their health data. This leads to profound privacy concerns, with instances of data being sold or shared without explicit consent. Once data is shared, it's often challenging to revoke access or ensure its deletion. Compounding these issues are security deficiencies, as centralized databases are more susceptible to unauthorized alteration of records. Despite significant regulatory pressure from frameworks like HIPAA, healthcare organizations still struggle with adequate data protection.

Web3 principles offer a robust antidote to these systemic flaws, particularly through decentralization, cryptographic security, and true user ownership. Decentralization, primarily powered by blockchain technology, means data is stored across multiple nodes in a distributed ledger network, eliminating single points of failure. The immutability inherent in blockchain ensures that once data is recorded, it cannot be altered or deleted, creating an unchangeable audit trail that enhances trust and accountability. This distributed nature makes it incredibly difficult for malicious actors to compromise the entire system, significantly enhancing security.

Radical Market Transparency

The first half of the belief: Radical transparency is a philosophy and practice of openness where all healthcare market data, processes, and outcomes are made available to everyone, fostering a culture of direct and honest communication. It goes beyond typical transparency by striving for full and immediate access to information, allowing for greater alignment, opportunity, and value creation.

With Personal Data Sovereignty

Elevate Health strikes a balance between market transparency and personal data sovereignty. Web3 champions user ownership and control. Tools such as Self-Sovereign Identity (SSI) empower individuals to create and manage their digital identities without relying on centralized authorities. Patients store their personal medical history in digital wallets and selectively present it to doctors, health systems, and other service providers. In addition, smart contracts can be set up to automate data access, permissions and data sharing rules based on the individual's preferences. In this way, Web3 technology can enable granular control to patients, allowing them to grant and revoke access to specific data elements for particular periods or purposes. These theoretical underpinnings allow Elevate Health 2050 to develop a transformative data architecture for healthcare markets. New secure Personal Health Records (PHRs) built on Web3 will enable patients to have unparalleled control over their complete medical history, accessible from various providers, with seamless interoperability between different healthcare systems, all underpinned by immutable audit trails of data access and modifications.

Consent management becomes transparent and auditable, particularly for data sharing in clinical trials and research, with the potential for incentivized data sharing, where individuals could receive cryptocurrency for contributing anonymized data. Beyond patient data, Web3 can revolutionize supply chain management for pharmaceuticals, tracking the provenance of drugs to combat counterfeiting and ensuring the authenticity and integrity of medical supplies. Even decentralized clinical trials can benefit from secure and transparent management of trial data, as well as enhanced patient privacy for participants. Web3 tools offer a truly transformative solution for personal health data privacy and autonomy, moving us beyond the vulnerabilities of centralized systems. They promise enhanced security through cryptographic methods and immutability, unprecedented patient control through self-sovereign identity and smart contracts, greater transparency in data sharing, and improved interoperability across the fragmented healthcare ecosystem.

We plan to use Web3 and blockchain technology to implement this belief directly into the Elevate Health 2050 infrastructure. This will allow the Elevate health market to deliver several inherent advantages, including.

- **Users are stakeholders, not products:** Web3 transforms engagement through transparent value-sharing.

- **Ownership economics reshape participation:** Incentives drive community involvement.
- **Pseudonymity enables merit-based reputation:** Systems reward expertise.
- **Protocol loyalty creates anti-fragile networks:** Building resilient systems.
- **Value capture shifts to participants:** Rewarding contributions.
- **Transparent governance builds trust at scale:** Ensuring accountability.
- **Portable identity enables cross-platform reputation:** Track records are not siloed.

The potential for a patient-centric health data infrastructure that combines Radical Market Transparency and Personal Data Sovereignty is immense. Elevate Health 2050 aims to usher in an era where complete transparency fosters trust, while balancing the complexities of healthcare costs, access, and quality in pursuit of our shared values. Simultaneously, individuals in Elevate Health are empowered to manage their personal health data and information. We understand this ideal will be challenging to implement and will encourage continued research, development, and collaboration to overcome the existing challenges and fully realize the benefits of these innovative technologies for a more secure and empowering future of health data.

Foundational belief #3: Race to the Top for Health

Anthropic, a leading AI safety and research company, has proposed a "Race to the Top" strategy for the responsible development of AI. This approach emphasizes leading by example, fostering collaboration, and promoting transparency to encourage the entire AI field to prioritize safety and ethics, instead of solely focusing on out-competing others. In an interview with Time magazine, Amodei framed the "Race to the Top" as an essential strategy linked to Anthropic's competitive approach. He described voluntarily constraining the release of more powerful AI models until adequate safety measures are developed, thereby pressuring competitors to adopt similar standards. Amodei clarified the goal is not adversarial but collaborative: "We're not trying to say we're the good guys and the others are the bad guys... We're trying to pull the ecosystem in a direction where everyone can be the good guy." (Time, 2024). This highlights Anthropic's aim to shift the industry's focus towards collective safety responsibility. Inspired by Anthropic's approach, Elevate Health seeks to apply this "Race to the Top" framework as a third foundational belief, guiding members toward a future where innovation and patient well-being are paramount.

Elevate Health will leverage the "Race to the Top" ideals to foster collaboration and transparency within the healthcare industry. By encouraging the sharing of knowledge and best practices, we accelerate the development of innovative solutions, leading to earlier diagnoses, more accurate assessments, and optimized treatments. This collaborative environment will also help reduce health disparities by mitigating biases in healthcare algorithms and ensuring equitable access to care for all populations. Imagine a future where the benefits of AI-driven healthcare are accessible to everyone, regardless of their background or location.

Applying a "Race to the Top" strategy in healthcare innovation holds immense promise for accelerating progress and improving patient care. By leading with our values, fostering collaboration, and promoting transparency, we can create a healthcare system that prioritizes safety, ethics, and equity. While challenges remain in ensuring the responsible development and deployment of AI-driven healthcare solutions, the potential benefits are undeniable. Elevate Health is committed to driving this positive change and shaping a brighter future for healthcare.

Three Perspectives on the Elevate Health Community:

While it is valuable to establish the Elevate Health Community's shared values and beliefs, we also find the discussion somewhat abstract. To paint a more nuanced understanding, we introduce three example community members: Heather, Paul & Andy. We hope getting to know these hypothetical members will help illustrate how the Elevate Health market improves the health and wellness of individuals.

Heather Healthcare

Heather Healthcare, a 35-year-old, is a dedicated nurse. She works at an academic medical center. She represents the frontline professional caregivers navigating the existing healthcare system every day. As a practicing nurse, Heather's focus is on optimizing patient care and coordination, while her personal health status enables her to prioritize general wellness.

She starts her day by helping her two boys get off to school, and then Heather heads into the healthcare system, where she is a Med/Surg nurse. On the weekends, Heather spends time with her husband and young family. As a professional, Heather is motivated by improving efficiency in patient care, reducing administrative friction, and ensuring comprehensive support for her patients and their families. She values convenience and preventative health. Heather has professional and personal pain points. On the work front, Fragmented patient data, communication silos between providers, and a lack of tools to easily coordinate complex care plans. In her personal life, Healthier struggles to find time for self-care and accessing preventative health resources. In the Elevate

Health Community, Heather is seeking robust, integrated tools, support services, and platforms that enable seamless communication among patients, caregivers, and providers. She is seeking tools that automate coordination and provide clear visualization of the patient journey, enabling her to optimize her workflow and prevent burnout.

Andy Armstrong

Andy is also 35 years old, but unlike Heather, he works at an outpatient imaging center company with sites across the US. Andy represents the entrepreneurial spirit driving the Elevate Health market and helps bring into focus the perspective of the hardworking service providers to the healthcare industry. Andy's professional focus is on delivering a great experience to every patient and employee, while also generating a fair return for his investors. He doesn't think much about his health. Andy occasionally works out by jogging, but he lacks discipline. Andy starts his day by working out and having breakfast with his teenage boys before heading to his office downtown. On weekends, he typically drives to sporting events with his sons or grabs a quick round of golf with friends.

In his job, Andy is driven by the desire to create a high-impact, profitable business that disrupts the status quo. One of Andy's biggest challenges is navigating regulatory hurdles, securing funding in a risk-averse industry, and integrating new technology with established healthcare infrastructure. He also faces the challenge of engaging healthy populations in preventative services. He is particularly interested in developing tools for individuals who are "worried well" and those with low-risk scores, who are interested in being proactive. On the personal front, Andy is not taking care of himself because he's too busy. In the Elevate Health Community, Andy needs clear regulatory pathways and a market environment that values innovative, data-driven solutions for personalized health.

Paul Patient

Paul is also 35 and works as a middle management "knowledge worker" in the healthcare industry. He is an accountant for a large insurance company. As a busy executive, Paul's focus is on doing good work and getting a promotion or maybe a raise. Paul doesn't think much about his health. He tries to exercise but never really sticks with anything. Paul begins his day by driving into work, listening to his podcasts and heading into his office in the suburbs.. On the weekends.

Paul is largely unmotivated by health concerns, as he feels fine. His primary motivations are convenience and minimizing disruption to his work and social life. The lack of symptoms means he doesn't see the need for healthcare intervention. Paul needs the Elevate Health Community to proactively identify his health risks and present helpful information in an accessible and non-threatening manner, helping him understand his health needs. We will return to follow these three example members over the next several chapters of the book.

Summary

Elevate Health has ambitious goals to elevate health to a higher priority, above political, cultural, and religious debates. This will only be accomplished with a large community of passionate and hard-working people working toward the same vision. In this chapter, we outline the initial versions of shared health values and foundational beliefs to guide this community. The vision is for the Elevate Health Community to grow into an open community with the characteristics of successful bootstrapped projects like WordPress. As we add members, we expect to monitor our shared health values and foundational beliefs continually. They may be updated and revised as needed. However, the goal is to develop long-lasting, shared values and foundational beliefs that change infrequently, serving to ground us in the knowledge that we all share these core ideals. From this source of shared strength, the Elevate Health community is then strong enough to engage in broad debates and test diverse ideas related to how best to implement, allocate, and regulate health. These trials and test projects become a source of learning and are not nearly as fear-inducing or threatening.

Chapter 5: Patients and Caregivers

Life is simple, but we insist on making it complicated.
– Confucius

As discussed in the first four chapters, Health markets are large and complicated. Yet in this chapter, we argue that while health markets are complex, the core healthcare transaction can be simplified into one essential relationship, between a patient and their caregiver. This insight enables Elevate Health to align all its community benefits with a focus on enhancing the patient/caregiver experience.

Every Member a "Patient"

Elevate Health 2050 is primarily designed to benefit its Individual Members. All members are patients; therefore, we start by focusing on providing healthcare services and tools to help members improve their health and wellness. We envision a

Personal Wellness AI-Coach as a guide to help members access the most valuable resources in the Elevate Health Community. All Members are granted free access to the Personal Wellness AI-Coach upon joining. The details of this core product are intentionally not specified here. It will leverage emerging capabilities from the AI, Web3 and Biotech innovation waves, but the specific implementation details will evolve and change over time. Instead, we present the vision for a suite of personal health services and tools designed to benefit members and facilitated by a dedicated AI-Coach.

A few key capabilities of the Personal Wellness AI-Coach:

- Designed to help Members understand their potential, set achievable health goals, and identify resources to support their success. It is 100% focused on the individual member and optimizing their health. This is inherently different than commercial AIs optimized for the entire population and often owned by large corporations.
- Tracks the Members' health preferences, beliefs, favorite physicians, and preferred news sources, ensuring this context is utilized when

the member interacts with caregivers, AI tools, future public health utilities, and all other Elevate Health market participants.

- Maintains a secure & encrypted repository of all personal health records for each Member, including conditions, goals, actions, tools, utilities, medications, labs, procedures, doctors, other caregivers, as well as how their health metrics have improved or deteriorated over time.

Imagine having an empathic nurse-like AI as your personal health coach, always with you. It follows your instructions and helps you to understand your choices and set realistic and achievable goals. This personal wellness coach has access to your complete medical records, but also recalls that you prefer to see your primary care doctor virtually, but your dermatologist in person. It has learned what types of incentives motivate you and uses this knowledge to develop fun and interactive personal health games that motivate you to make progress toward your goals over time. Most importantly, the Personal Wellness AI-Coach is designed to optimize the Member's health and wellness.

Cargiver Member Benefits

While the primary focus of Elevate Health 2050 will be on individuals, we expect many of our Members will also elect to contribute their skills and abilities to serve as caregivers. For some, if they are a physician, nurse or counselor, this will be easy. However, we will seek ways to involve as many members as possible in contributing care for others in the Elevate Health Community. As we age, our personal networks naturally become smaller and less engaged. For many, this leads to a need for human connection, fulfillment, and meaning. Simultaneously, many of our members' care needs will not require advanced degrees and extensive training. Instead, Members will need support, companionship, and assistance in the typical activities of daily living.

To encourage and empower members to become caregivers, Elevate Health plans to offer a second product named "Top of Calling." This product is specifically designed to assist with caregiver productivity. It will also leverage AI and Web3 to serve Members based on their qualifications, capacity, and interests in providing care in the community. The "Top of Calling" brand is meant to signal the purpose of the tool. Many incumbent organizations have established programs designed to help providers practice at the "Top of their License." While this has been a useful concept, we believe it focuses too much on the transactional and billing aspects of healthcare. Most physicians, nurses, and other caregivers did not enter a career in healthcare to maximize billing or earn the most income. Therefore, the Top of Calling caregiver product helps members realize their true calling, in whatever form that may take.

The two products will be intrinsically linked together. It is our vision that the Personal Wellness AI-Coach may help the Member discover opportunities to find meaning and purpose in providing care to other members. When a Member shows interest in caregiving, they are provided access to Top of Calling. This will be true for licensed healthcare workers, as well as non-traditional caregivers. For instance, members with personal experience navigating a cancer diagnosis (aka cancer survivors) may be willing to share experiences and provide empathic listening to other members earlier in their battle against the disease. This compassionate caregiving role has been underappreciated, and Elevate Health intends to foster connections between members. To illustrate how unlicensed caregivers can benefit the community, we look to the Friendship Bench success story.

The Friendship Bench

Zimbabwe is not a rich, developed country. They have approximately 15 million people and, unfortunately, only about 20 trained and licensed psychiatrists. This is a tough challenge, but necessity is the mother of invention. The Zimbabwe Ministry of Health needed to find a solution because they were in such desperate need. They developed a low-cost program for psychosocial support, known as the Friendship Bench. This program used elderly women with time on their hands to sit on the bench and listen with empathy. Of course, they're not psychiatrists, and therefore can't diagnose disease or provide clinical treatment. However, the simple act of listening and connecting with people and offering basic empathic messages such as “I care about you,” “I want you to feel better,” or “Let's look to see if our community already offers programs that could help you”- can have significant positive benefits.

Last year in Zimbabwe, 60,000 people received this service, which is very low-cost, approaching free. In addition, the Friendship Bench has been studied extensively, with over a hundred peer-reviewed papers describing how it works, why it works, and validating its outcomes. Participants in the Friendship Bench program were shown to be better off at 3 and 6-month follow-up points, according to a range of indicators, including fear, anger, and sleep patterns, compared to those who received therapy from a community mental health nurse or psychologist. The surprising results were that both patients and volunteer caregivers felt more supported and connected to their community. In this way, the Friendship Bench has been a genuine win-win program. The people seeking treatment are heard and supported, while the caregiving role provides a sense of purpose for the volunteers. This is an excellent example of how some of the best innovations don't require massive venture capital investment, and they often don't need FDA approval. Instead, they identify available resources within the community and align interests to create a program that benefits both the caregiver and the patient.

The Power of Positive Incentives

Once all members of the Elevate Health Community have a Personal Wellness AI-Coach, we can begin to leverage the power of positive incentives in combination with our shared values and beliefs. As the community is not yet formed, we make some assumptions about the types of health goals our members will have and, therefore, the healthcare needs they will require. Yet we believe these assumptions to be realistic. We project that a high percentage of our members will have one or more chronic diseases, including Diabetes, COPD, Kidney disease, and Heart Disease. This is likely because, according to a study published by the US Ceneter for Disease Control & Prevention (CDC), more than 75% of all Americans over the age of 35 have at least one chronic disease. Each Member will interact with their Personal Wellness AI-Coach to identify goals and improve their health. However, for those with chronic disease, we expect this to often result in one of three broad activities:

1. Work to comply with existing treatments and recommendations
2. Seek additional healthcare services to manage their disease more effectively and reduce symptoms and or reduce future risks.

3. Strive to improve their health and wellness in a novel direction due to personal interest or in pursuit of a desired goal.

In this way, although each Member will have complete freedom over their health goals, we can forecast that engaged Members will increase their utilization of healthcare services and expand the overall market. This is important as we do not expect early Members to abandon their existing healthcare services. Instead, we expect members to add Elevate Health, an adjunct health system, in addition to existing systems. Innovations from the 3 waves will allow our Personal Wellness AI-Coach to effectively navigate the range of potential service offerings available through the Elevate Health Community benefits. There will be many options available to members, including:

- Free health services and educational content provided to the Elevate Health Community by a High-Margin Organization as a part of their 10% reinvestment program.
- High-Margin healthcare products and services. These will often be cutting-edge, innovative healthcare treatments and procedures. They

will require the Member to pay either directly or through an insurance arrangement. However, the benefits of the services relative to Low-Margin alternatives will be clearly explained by the Personal Wellness AI-Coach to allow the Member as much choice as possible. While the profit margins are high, Members understand that 10% of their payment will be reinvested to help others in the community. Furthermore, the cost is fully transparent, and payment is delivered to the care provider within 7 days following the service. More information about this healthcare settlement service in the next chapter.

- Low-Margin healthcare products and services. These are often established and common healthcare treatments and procedures. They require the Member to pay either directly or through an insurance arrangement, but members are confident that the profit margins are less than 15%. Furthermore, the cost is fully transparent, and payment is made to the care provider within 7 days of the service.
- Peer & Community Services. These offerings are not clinical, but like the Friendship Bench, they can be highly effective. Some peer and

community services are free, and others are qualified as low-margin. The benefits of these services, as well as how they complement or take the place of other services, are clearly explained to allow the Member as much choice as possible.

Members will have the opportunity to use these service offerings within the Elevate Health Community. There is no requirement, and all member engagement is voluntary. As members select from the above options, they will begin to experience a health market aligned around values and beliefs with Members at the center. When they choose a High-margin service, that organization will reinvest 10% of the cost as resources (in-kind services, research, cash, etc.) to support public health initiatives. In this way, the market infrastructure will grow and improve over time.

One of the key lessons from bootstrapping companies is to use the long-term time horizon as a competitive advantage. The Elevate Health Market is designed to be stable and resilient, providing high-quality healthcare at all scales. It does not need to grow to any size to deliver value to its members. Yet it is also not constrained. As required, Elevate Health can quickly expand to provide support to individuals who have lost healthcare coverage and require immediate assistance. If Elevate Health is to navigate the potential coming crisis to emerge as the best global health market in 2050, this resiliency is a critical aspect. Over time and at their own pace, Members will transition to trust the Elevate Health market for more of their healthcare services. Over 5, 10, or 25 years, the Elevate Health Community will organically develop and grow from the bottom up. In this way, we allow the market to be "bootstrapped" to meet the needs of its members.

Onboarding Our Illustrative Personas:

We can now return to the personas introduced in the last chapter to examine the initial onboarding member experience. As a part of the End Heart Disease Project, detailed later in Chapter 10, Heather, Andy, and Paul join the Elevate Health Community to get a free "Heart Health Calcium Screen." The community has a grant that funds this quick 30-minute diagnostic image screen for all members over 35 years of age.

The process works as follows: any interested person aged 35 or older simply completes a 3-question intake form, providing their name, phone number, and date of birth. Then they book an appointment for the screening. Within 24 hours after the screening, they are welcomed to the Elevate Health Community via text message by their new Personal Wellness AI-Coach. The onboarding is designed to be easy and fun. The AI-Coach's role is to learn about the member and assist them in clarifying and then working toward their goals. Using the calcium score, Elevate Health places each Member on one of two paths. If the Calcium Score is 0, the AI-Coach knows the Member is low risk for heart disease. It gives them this great news and asks if they have any other health and wellness goals. However, if the Calcium Score is positive, the Wellness Coach knows the member has some existing heart disease. It uses the exact CA score to estimate the severity of disease and helps the member understand that heart disease typically develops slowly over many decades. The bad news is that the Member has some evidence of Heart Disease, but the good news is that by catching it early, they have several effective treatment options. Once the AI-Coach educates the member and takes some additional key data points, such as "do they smoke?"

and "what is their height & weight?" and "have they ever had a cholesterol test?" The member has the option to find an appropriate physician independently or use one of the options available in the Elevate Health 2050 Community.

Heather Healthcare:

Heather hears about the offer from a coworker. She is curious about the screen and also wants to experience the Personal Wellness AI-Coach for herself. Her coworker didn't have heart disease, but she has already lost five pounds with the "coach," and looks great. Heather gets the Heart Health Calcium Screen and is excited to review the results with the Personal Wellness AI-Coach. She has a Calcium score of 0, which is the best score possible. It means she has no signs of heart disease, and doesn't have to worry about that for about 10 years. As Heather interacts with the AI, she sets some personal goals but is most excited about the "Top of Calling" added functionality. She begins to learn about the many new options open to her in the Elevate Health Community.

Paul Patient

Paul's wife encourages him to get the Heart Health Screen. He goes to get the test, but unlike Heather,

Paul isn't excited about the idea. He feels fine and hates to take time out of his weekend to get the test. Although it only takes 30 minutes, he avoids it for a few months until he finally makes the effort to go. When Paul gets his results, his Calcium score is 75. This indicates that he has heart disease and his body is using Calcium to repair damage along the inside of his blood vessels.

When the Personal AI-Wellness Coach gives Paul these results, it also provides him with an introductory video explaining the evidence of heart disease and informing him about available treatment options. The AI Coach has unlimited patience and happily answers all of Paul's questions and helps him understand his alternatives. The AI Coach's motivation is to maximize Paul's personal health and wellness. From this point of view, it supports Paul in processing this scary test result and encourages him to either talk to his current doctor or begin a relationship with one of the Elevate Health 2050 Caregivers. Unfortunately, Paul is not yet ready to face his potential heart disease. He watches the videos and asks several questions of the AI Coach, but ultimately, Paul elects not to tell his wife and to continue ignoring his health issues. He is unmotivated and slightly paralyzed by the fear he feels when thinking about his results. He tells himself that he has plenty of time, and with no symptoms, he tries to forget about the concerning news. Unfortunately, this response is typical. Paul "feels fine" and is not convinced of the necessity of preventative care.

Andy Armstrong

Andy reads about the Heart Health Calcium Screen and is interested in learning more about the program. He is not concerned about his health, but he is interested in learning about how the technology works as he thinks there may be a business opportunity for his company. Andy gets the Heart Health Calcium Screen and is curious to test out the AI system for himself. His Calcium score is 5, which indicates he has the beginning of heart disease. When the Personal AI-Wellness Coach gives Andy these results, it also provides him with an introductory video explaining the evidence of heart disease and informing him about the available treatment options. Andy is intrigued by the AI-Coach and asks lots of questions to understand his options fully. The AI-Coach's motivation is to maximize Andy's health and wellness. From this point of view, it supports Andy in processing this new data point. It encourages him to either talk to his current doctor or begin a relationship with one of the Elevate Health 2050 Caregivers. Andy brings up the topic with his primary care doctor and starts taking a daily Statin medication. Andy chats with the AI-Coach from time to time, but he does not set any new health goals at this time.

Ellie Engagement (new persona)

We are introducing a 4th persona: Ellie. Ellie is also 35 and works as a middle management “knowledge worker” in the healthcare industry. She is a software engineer for a large pharmaceutical company. Like Paul and Andy, she is primarily focused on her work and family. Ellie has never worried much about her health. She tries to eat well and exercise, but she lacks motivation. Ellie rides the subway to work in a large US city. She is married with no children. On the weekends, she enjoys listening to live music with friends and traveling. Ellie does not think about her health much and feels fine. Her primary motivations are convenience and minimizing disruption to her work and social life. The lack of symptoms means she doesn't see the need for healthcare intervention. Ellie needs the Elevate Health Community to proactively identify her health risks and present useful information in an accessible manner, helping her understand her health needs.

Ellie learns about the program from her older sister, who asks her to please get the Heart Health Calcium Screen. She does it because it's free and there is a screening location conveniently located near her office. When Ellie gets her results, her Calcium score is 75. This indicates that she has heart disease and her body is using Calcium to try to repair damage along the inside of her blood vessels. When the Personal Wellness AI-Coach gives Ellie these results, it also provides her with an introductory video explaining the evidence of heart disease and informing her about the available treatment options. The AI-Coach has unlimited patience and happily answers all of her questions. It even conducts a 3-way question and answer session with Ellie and her husband. The AI-Coach's motivation is to maximize Ellie's personal health and wellness. From this point of view, it supports Ellie in processing this scary test result. It encourages her to either talk to her current doctor or begin a relationship with one of the Elevate Health Caregivers. Unlike Paul, Ellie is motivated by the results of her screening. She is pragmatic and understands the gravity of the elevated score, choosing to trust the AI-Coach's guidance. Ellie finds a

Cardiologist through the Elevate Health Community and begins to focus on improving her health. She is prescribed daily Statin medication, begins doing yoga 3 times per week, and sets a goal to begin eating a healthier diet. Ellie represents a Member with significant underlying risk who chooses to engage with the Elevate Health Market.

Summary

Elevate Health 2025 simplifies the complex healthcare market to the core patient-caregiver relationship. This allows us to start providing value to Members through two primary interfaces. First, we give all Members a Personal =Wellness AI-Coach. This allows the community to cut through all the typical paperwork and endless data entry and jump directly to giving the Members an empathic personal health coach, immediately providing value. Onboarding is simple, short, and intuitive. Elevate Health meets its Members where they are and allows them to set the pace of change. This AI-Coach is complemented with our caregiver productivity tool: Top of Calling. It enables the community to make connections between patients and caregivers in a mutually beneficial manner.

Health markets todfay are far too complex and confusing to navigate. By limiting the Elevate Health Community interface to these two products, we dramatically simplify the member experience facilitating meaningful connections.   Finally, the Elevate Health Market is designed to be stable and resilient, providing high-quality healthcare at any scale. It does not need to grow to any size to deliver value to its members. Yet it is also not constrained. Over time and at their own pace, members will transition to trust the Elevate Health market for more of their healthcare services. Over 5, 10, or 25 years, the Elevate Health Community will organically develop and grow from the bottom up.

Chapter 6: Market Infrastructure

The future is already here – it's just not evenly distributed.

- *William Gibson*

In previous chapters, we outlined the vision for Elevate Health 2050 to align around shared values and foundational beliefs. We also illustrated how a patient-centric system could function. This chapter aims to address the most common objections to the Elevate Health concept. We discuss the infrastructure required to deliver healthcare independent of traditional centralized authorities.

Our healthcare system is immense and entrenched. It may be difficult to imagine how this incumbent system could be replaced without the US government as the central regulator and primarily funder. We have all grown up in a society that provides healthcare primarily through a centralized government. The US has the most market-based healthcare system in the world, and yet it is still 50% funded and regulated mainly by the federal government. In other countries, the federal government provides a larger share of healthcare services. If we are to elevate health above politics, we must address how a new healthcare market can be established, regulated, and funded independently of centralized authorities, such as governments or employers.

This chapter will confront these crucial questions head-on, revealing the innovative market infrastructure that makes the Elevate Health vision not only possible but robust and resilient. We describe how our shared foundational beliefs #2 Radical Market Transparency and Personal Data Sovereignty and #3 Race to the Top of Health provide the infrastructure powered by Web3 technologies to address these concerns.

Trust in Government at an All-Time Low

In 1958, during the last high period, approximately 75% of Americans trusted the government. This confidence in elected officials and government institutions began to decline in the 1980s. Declines in trust were due to a combination of dissatisfaction with governmental accountability and skepticism about the competency of institutions. Gallup's historical polling data corroborate this pattern, providing additional granular detail. In 1972, according to Gallup, combined trust levels (those expressing either "great deal" or "fair amount" of trust) reached 75%. By 2024, this had fallen to 37%, with particularly sharp declines evident in the period following the 2007 financial crisis. The data shows that while trust fluctuated in earlier decades, consistently low levels characterize the post-2007 period. Current data shows that 35% of self-declared Democrats express trust in the federal government, compared with only 11% of self-declared Republicans.

The decline in trust is not confined to the United States but is part of a broader global trend. Pew Research compiled data on developed countries shows that between 2006 and 2012, confidence in government fell by at least six percentage points in 18 of the 34 OECD member nations. Ireland experienced the steepest drop, with confidence plummeting from 63% in 2006 to 35% in 2012, a decline of 28 percentage points over six years. European data shows particularly concerning trends, with data from the United Nations indicating trust in political parties in European Union countries has remained consistently low, hovering between 15-20% on average between 2000 and 2019. The decline in trust in government has significant implications for policy implementation and compliance with government directives. Research consistently shows that higher levels of trust are associated with greater willingness to comply with laws, pay taxes, and support government policies. The sustained low levels of trust documented in this research, therefore, represent a significant challenge to effective governance.

Corporations Treat People as Products

The promise of powerful AI is often packaged with a hidden cost: the leverage of personal data for profit and platform lock-in. Companies like OpenAI, Meta, Amazon, Microsoft, and Google are racing to develop dominant AI models to use this power to monetize their platforms. The most straightforward path to profitability is through the strategic use of personal data, creating tension between the benefits of personalization and the risks of privacy infringement. This dynamic is illustrated by the user response to new features like OpenAI's "Memory" function for ChatGPT.

The introduction of OpenAI's Memory feature for ChatGPT has been met with mixed user feedback. On one hand, the feature offers enhanced personalization, allowing the AI to recall past interactions, preferences, and details. This is achieved as the system learns and stores details such as their boss's name or a preferred coding language, over time. This functionality is a major convenience, saving users the effort of repeating themselves in every new chat. It fosters a more natural, continuous dialogue and enables the generation of more relevant and customized responses, enhancing the overall user experience. However, these benefits come with significant privacy and control concerns. A central point of contention is data retention and deletion. Users have voiced skepticism about whether "deleted" information truly disappears, leading to fears that their data may persist longer than claimed. Another concern centers on the automatic nature of memory saving. Some users are dissatisfied with memories being saved by default, arguing for more granular control over what information is stored. This lack of transparency and user control has raised serious questions about OpenAI's commitment to ethical AI practices, especially in the wake of the dissolution of its superalignment team, which was responsible for ensuring the safety and ethics of advanced AI.

The automatic and persistent accumulation of personal data through features like Memory creates a significant risk of user lock-in. As a user's digital history, preferences, and details become deeply embedded within one AI platform, the switching costs to another service become prohibitively high. This creates a data moat that makes it incredibly difficult for competing services to gain traction, further entrenching the market dominance of a few large players. Users become tied to a specific AI ecosystem not just by habit, but by the sheer volume of personal information they would have to rebuild elsewhere, a process that is both time-consuming and often impossible. The current trajectory of AI development, driven by a handful of large corporations, seems to prioritize user engagement and data accumulation over ethical safeguards and user autonomy. This approach not only threatens individual privacy but also stifles innovation by creating monopolistic market dynamics.

This is why Elevate Health's belief in Personal Data Sovereignty is foundational. Elevate Health markets do not ask Members to "trust us" to keep personal data secure. Rather, we architect Personal Data Sovereignty into the foundations of the market. In Elevate Health, Members' data truly belongs to each member—not to a corporation. This ensures Members have 100% control over their information, deciding what is shared, when it is shared, and with whom. This approach shifts the power and authority from the platform to the individual, ensuring that the benefits of personalization can be enjoyed without sacrificing privacy or becoming locked into a single ecosystem. By building systems where data sovereignty is a core feature, Elevate Health fosters a community that aligns personal data sovereignty with innovation and value creation.

Trust through Radical Transparency & Personal Data Sovereignty

Elevate Health replaces reliance on untrustworthy central governments and corporations with a community aligned around shared values and beliefs. Our second foundational belief—Radical Market Transparency, combined with Personal Data Sovereignty—is designed to build confidence in the accuracy of Elevate Health data while fiercely protecting personal privacy through advanced encryption technologies.

We leverage a key tenet of Web3, decentralization, to deliver on this core belief. Instead of a single, central database that serves as an attractive target for hackers, we use Web3 technology to distribute data across a network of computers or nodes. This design eliminates the single points of failure that make current systems so vulnerable to cyberattacks and data breaches. By dispersing medical records and other sensitive information, the system becomes more resilient and secure. This is akin to replacing a single, high-value target with thousands of smaller, fortified outposts, making a coordinated attack more difficult than the data is worth.

The encryption layer in our Web3 infrastructure provides multiple levels of protection that traditional healthcare systems simply cannot match. In traditional healthcare systems, data breaches can result in loss of patient trust and significant financial damages. However, with our advanced encryption approach, even in the unlikely event of a security incident, the encrypted data remains unreadable and therefore useless to unauthorized parties. This level of protection not only ensures compliance with healthcare regulations but also provides peace of mind to patients who can trust that military-grade encryption protocols safeguard their most sensitive personal information. Furthermore, the foundational principle of immutability ensures a new level of trust and accountability. Medical data stored on a blockchain, a core technology of Web3, cannot be altered or deleted once it's recorded. This creates a permanent, unchangeable audit trail of every interaction, from a doctor's diagnosis to a prescription refill. For the patient, this means their medical history is reliable and tamper-proof. For the provider, it means a secure record that can't be falsified. For the payer, it enhances the ability to fight fraud and ensures transparency in billing and claims processing.

Member Empowerment

We empower individuals, giving them user control and data ownership through sophisticated encryption mechanisms. In Elevate Health markets, Members are no longer just data points in a corporate ledger; they become the owners of their own medical history. Within the Personal Wellness AI-Coach product,

Elevate Health provides each Member with a secure & encrypted repository of all health records, including conditions, medications, labs, procedures, doctors, other caregivers, as well as how their health metrics have improved or deteriorated over time. The AI-Coach assists the Member in managing the cryptographic keys to unlock and share this data as desired. This gives each individual the power to selectively grant access to a new doctor, a specialist, or a researcher for a limited time, fundamentally changing the patient-caregiver dynamic and returning power to the patient.

The cryptographic key system is an inherent aspect of the Web3 market infrastructure and represents a revolutionary advancement in data security. Unlike traditional password-based systems that can be compromised through various attack vectors, cryptographic keys provide mathematically secure access control. Each Member possesses a unique set of encryption keys that are virtually impossible to replicate or forge. These keys enable patients to maintain complete control over who can access their health information, when they can access it, and for how long. The encryption ensures that even healthcare providers can only view the specific data that patients have explicitly authorized them to see.

In this way, Elevate Health addresses one of today's most significant privacy concerns, the unauthorized sharing or selling of patient data. With traditional systems, once a healthcare organization has access to patient information, there are limited technical barriers preventing misuse of that data. However, with our Web3 approach, patient data remains encrypted even when shared with authorized parties. Caregivers and healthcare organizations receive temporary decryption keys that allow them to access only the specific information needed for treatment, and these keys automatically expire after the predetermined period.

Granular control is made possible through a Web3 innovation called "smart contracts." These are self-executing agreements with the terms of the agreement directly written into code. The AI-Coach collaborates with the Member to determine their personal data sharing preferences. Then, the AI can handle all of the complexity related to developing smart contracts to automate data access and sharing rules while maintaining the highest levels of encryption security. For example, a patient could ask their Personal Wellness AI-Coach to set up a smart contract that automatically grants their primary care physician access to their fitness tracker data for the duration of a treatment plan but revokes it afterward. The smart contract ensures that all data exchanges are encrypted end-to-end, creating an audit trail of access while maintaining the confidentiality of the information being shared. This not only gives patients fine-tuned control but also streamlines administrative processes, reducing paperwork and human error while respecting patient preferences and maintaining the highest security standards.

Radical Market Transparency

Elevate Health pairs this Personal Data Sovereignty with Radical Market Transparency. Healthcare markets have been difficult to understand and opaque. Patients are frequently left in the dark about costs, quality, and outcomes. The lack of clear information creates an environment where inefficiencies thrive, and consumer trust erodes. Elevate Health turns this on its head with our Radical Market Transparency belief. We make 100% of all healthcare market data, processes, and outcomes available to the public. By aggregating data into groups of at least 100 Members, we ensure anonymity for individuals while empowering market participants with the transparency and information needed to make informed decisions. This fundamental shift from secrecy to openness has the potential to transform healthcare markets for the better.

A central pain point in the current healthcare system is the convoluted and delayed billing process. Elevate Health directly addresses this issue by demanding full transparency on costs and offering payment processing and settlement in 7 days for a 1% fee. Organizations are required to provide transparency to Elevate Health as a part of agreeing to our shared values and beliefs. However, they are not required to use the payment processing and settlement service. This approach allows Elevate Health to eliminate the surprise bills and complex Explanations of Benefits (EOBs) that plague patients, replacing them with a straightforward, clear understanding of what a service will cost. For providers, this translates to predictable revenue streams and reduced administrative overhead. Many estimates suggest that Revenue Cycle Management and claims processing account for up to 10% of the total healthcare costs. This streamlined process benefits all parties, moving the focus from administrative battles to providing quality care.

Beyond pricing, Radical Market Transparency brings much-needed clarity to the quality and effectiveness of care. Transparent outcome reporting for services, providers, and treatments allows patients to compare options based on real-world results, not just marketing materials. For example, a Member facing a surgical procedure could easily access data on the success rates, complication rates, and recovery times for different surgeons or hospitals. Again, the Personal Wellness AI-Coach is well-suited to collect data from many options and help the Member evaluate what is best for them. This not only empowers Members to choose the best-performing providers but also incentivizes providers to continuously improve their outcomes. This public accountability drives a system-wide focus on excellence, ensuring that the highest standards of care become the norm, not the exception.

Tension Between For-Profit Organizations and Societal Good

As discussed in Chapter 3, the for-profit business model has been instrumental in driving innovation and improving efficiency in health markets. However, as the previous world order fractures, inherent tensions between profit-seeking goals and broader societal objectives have emerged. These firms, from large insurers and pharmacy benefit managers (PBMs) to hospitals and private equity-backed physician groups, operate under a fiduciary duty to maximize value for their shareholders. Regulatory changes have significantly influenced the participation of for-profit companies in expanding access to care. Telehealth, retail clinics, and managed care are prime examples. However, potential trade-offs exist between profit motives and equitable access in these new markets. For instance, telehealth providers might focus on patients with high-speed internet access and technological literacy, potentially excluding those in rural or underserved communities.

For-profit companies have been at the forefront of developing groundbreaking treatments and technologies. However, intellectual property patents, marketing practices, and pricing strategies can significantly impact the accessibility and affordability of these advancements. Consider the ethical implications of a company pricing a life-saving drug out of reach for most patients. Balancing profit motives with patient well-being requires a multifaceted approach. This includes promoting transparency in pricing, encouraging responsible marketing practices, and fostering a regulatory environment that incentivizes the development of affordable treatments. Additionally, fostering a culture of ethical research and development within for-profit companies is crucial to ensure patient needs remain paramount.

The public's frustration with these dynamics is palpable and has been increasingly visible, fueled by high-profile cases and the rising cost of care. The tragic murder of UnitedHealthcare CEO Brian Thompson in 2024 brought into sharp relief the widespread anger felt by many towards a healthcare system they perceive as uncaring and driven solely by financial gain.

A system that can harness the dynamism and resources of the market without sacrificing the core ethical responsibility of providing equitable and affordable care for all remains a key public policy challenge. As we navigate the transition to the

Intelligence Age, focusing on shared values is crucial for building a resilient and equitable healthcare system. By refining the message and creating a platform for dialogue, we will inspire collective action towards achieving this shared vision. This involves fostering a culture of ethical innovation within for-profit companies, implementing robust regulations that prioritize patient needs, and promoting collaboration across different sectors. Ultimately, the goal is to create a healthcare system that harnesses the power of innovation to improve the well-being of all members.

Elevate Health's 1st Foundational Belief redefines the categories of healthcare organizations. The old categories of "For-Profit" and "Non-Profit " are outdated and suggest a false dichotomy or false choice. These labels incorrectly imply that some organizations are working to "make money," and others are "helping people." This is inaccurate and unfair to both sides. Instead of using the organization's tax categories, we establish High-Margin and Low-Margin organizations. All health organizations with gross margins over 15% are defined as "High-Margin." Organizations delivering products and services with a gross margin less than

15% are described as "Low-Margin." This new framework allows the Elevate Health Community to require all High-Margin organizations then to invest at least 10% of their revenues back into the community, fostering trust through structured and transparent contributions.

Community 10% Re-Investment

This radical transparency is used as a powerful tool to align incentives and rebuild trust. By mandating High-Margin healthcare organizations publicly disclose how they contribute 10% of their revenue to public health initiatives, a clear connection is established between private success and public good. Furthermore, because Elevate Health is providing the settlement, it can enforce compliance. This visibility holds organizations accountable and highlights their commitment to the broader community, rather than solely focusing on profit margins. In this way, Elevate Health fosters a sense of shared responsibility, where highly profitable enterprises play a visible role in improving the health of the population they serve.

Ultimately, Radical Market Transparency engenders market participants to follow our third shard belief - and Race to the Top of Health. When all market data, from pricing to outcomes, is openly available, providers are motivated to not only improve their own performance but also to collaborate and share best practices. A hospital with an innovative procedure that leads to better outcomes would be incentivized to share its methods, knowing that it would contribute to a collective improvement in care and attract more patients seeking excellence. This constant cycle of innovation and collaboration, driven by transparent data, accelerates the development and adoption of new technologies and treatments. By making healthcare an open book, we can create a system that is more efficient, more equitable, and more focused on delivering the best possible outcomes for everyone.

Intellectual Property in an Abundant World

We are entering an age where no human intelligence will exist that isn't already commonly "known" within multiple AI models. Our expectation is that generalized intelligence poses a significant challenge to our current intellectual property (IP) framework. Over the next 25 years, there is a high probability that markets will need to account for the "commodization of IP assets." Established laws, legal precedent, and regulatory policies will need to be redesigned to accommodate the three waves of innovation in the Intelligence Age. Elevate Health 2050 must plan for a world where any human can easily recreate a song, a pharmaceutical compound, or a software program from scratch using AI. The core purpose of IP law is to encourage invention and discovery, but when new IP can be easily replicated, traditional IP law fails to serve this purpose. The key challenge lies in adapting a system designed for a world of scarcity and manual creation to one of abundance and automated replication.

IP Loophole: Clean Room Reverse Engineering

One of the most instructive historical examples of this challenge is the 1980s battle between Compaq and IBM. In a landmark case that established a new precedent for legal reverse engineering, Compaq became the first company to produce a portable IBM-compatible machine legally. They did this by using a meticulous "clean room design" to reverse engineer IBM's BIOS without violating copyright laws. This case provides a cautionary tale of how foundational technology is vulnerable despite existing IP protection.

The core challenge for Compaq was IBM's PC BIOS (Basic Input Output System), which was protected by copyright. The BIOS was the critical interface between the computer's software and hardware. Any company wanting to create a compatible machine had to replicate the BIOS's functionality. Companies like Eagle had already tried and failed, getting sued for directly copying IBM's code. The question for Compaq was how to create a functionally identical BIOS without infringing on IBM's copyright. They needed to understand what the program did, without ever looking at how it was done.

To achieve this, Compaq developed a "clean room" process to prevent any legal contamination. The solution involved two separate teams. First, the analysis team studied the IBM manuals and computers to understand exactly what functions the BIOS needed to accomplish. This team, which was "contaminated" with knowledge of IBM's design and code, could not legally write the software for Compaq. Rather, they documented the functional requirements, but not the code itself, and passes this detailed documentation to the implementation team. This second team of "clean" engineers, who had never seen the IBM manuals or code, wrote an entirely new BIOS from scratch, based solely on the functional specifications provided. In this way, Compaq did not violate IBM's IP protection and yet successfully developed a competitive product.

The results for Compaq were extraordinary. They successfully created a 95% IBM-compatible BIOS, and their first product, the Compaq Portable, hit the market in November 1982. The company anticipated $30 million in sales but instead raked in $111 million in its first year. By 1985, Compaq's sales had soared to $503 million, making it one of the fastest-growing companies in history. This success wasn't just a win for Compaq; it was a win for the entire PC industry, which was now free to innovate and compete without fear of copyright infringement. The legal precedent established by this case was profound. It affirmed the principle that you cannot copyright the functional requirements or behavior of software, only the specific implementation. The court recognized that reverse engineering for compatibility was a matter of Fair Use. The critical distinction was between looking at what a program does (its functional behavior) versus how it does it (its source code implementation). This legal clarity allowed Compaq to innovate by building a compatible system while still respecting IBM's right to its specific code. It created an environment where competition could flourish, even in a market dominated by a single player.

The clean room technique and the legal precedent it established will create new IP challenges in the Intelligence Age. Prior to the AI innovation wave, the clean room technique was feasible but capital and time-intensive. If a competitor wanted to reverse engineer a product protected by intellectual property, they had to hire two teams of experts. One was needed to document the specific functional requirements, and a second team was needed to build the new product to these requirements. While Compaq proved the process was possible, it was difficult to execute and only worth the cost for large market opportunities. However, using AI, these barriers have fallen dramatically. Elevate Health expects to see small teams of 2-3 people able to execute this process with the help of AI tools. This will have the effect of devaluing Intellectual Property and forever change competitive markets.

Intellectual Property in the Elevate Health 2050 Community

Intellectual Property laws and regulations must be updated for the Intelligence Age and the next world order. This is one of the first significant challenges to our existing status quo, but it will be one of many over the next several years. Instead of simply providing a proposed solution, we suggest that Elevate Health 2050 develop a methodology to define, evaluate, debate, and propose both challenges to the status quo (such as IP Laws) that can be used for all challenges in the transition to the new status quo optimized for the Intelligence Age. Elevate Health Community will define the challenge, evaluate it in terms of our shared values and beliefs, debate alternatives, and propose solutions designed to benefit the Members' health and wellness as much as possible.

In this case, we start by considering our 3rd value. According to Elevate Health Value #3: Aligned

Incentives and Innovation, the community must foster collaboration and innovation to optimize resources and deliver the best possible care. This value illustrates how protecting financial incentives for IP holders encourages the continuous pursuit of new discoveries and valuable innovation. For this reason, fair intellectual policy is essential to the overall Elevate Health community. This first value highlights the importance of IP protection, but does not resolve how the clean room loophole should be addressed..

To develop a new IP policy aligned to benefit the overall Elevate Health Community, we also consider Elevate Health's Community Belief #1: High and Low Margin Business Categories. Intellectual Property most often will be discovered and developed by a High-Margin organization. It is beneficial to the community overall to encourage the creation of new IP. Thus, when a new idea is discovered, by a Human or by an AI, they may use it to deliver a High-profit Margin health and wellness service without any other High-profit competition for a period of 5 years. This allows the creator to earn significant rewards for successfully developing valuable IP. However, we reduce the protected time from 20 to 5 years, but eliminate the IP enforcement role as the Elevate Health Community records the IP timing. This reduction in protected time decreases the IP asset value, as the cost of discovering and bringing a new concept to market is also decreasing by more than 4x. Of course, the High Margin organization would also make the standard 10%reinvestment in the community. This change to the IP protection policy is helpful, but not quite enough. We also need to consider Elevate Health Community Belief #3.

This third belief of the Elevate Health Community is the mindset of Race to the Top of Health. We believe in sharing knowledge and best practices to accelerate the adoption of innovation. To incorporate this ethos into the IP Policy, Low-margin "public health" services may use the IP after 3 years as long as they do not charge over 14.9% gross margins. For clarity: the policy makes two changes from the accepted standards in the US I world order. The first change shortens the IP protection period from 20 years under US law today to 5 years under the EH2050 policy. In addition, under EH2050, individuals and public health utilities are allowed to use the IP after 3 years. Both of these changes cause new inventions to receive sufficient rewards in the market to encourage continuous research and development. But they also more quickly turn the IP to a public good to encourage the Race to the Top culture. One can get a competitive advantage and sustain it over time only by continuously innovating and inventing.

The Market in Action: Reconnecting with Our Personas

We now turn to reconnect with the Key Personas in the Community. This helps ground the abstract policy discussion to the actual people getting healthcare. For each of the 4 personas, we discuss their lifetime trajectory with the Elevate Health 2050 market for the next 25 years. In the following four sections, we describe the persona's health span on Elevate Health, the age they died, and how they used the Community, if at all. We then explain the value of this persona and what we can learn from their fictional life trajectory.

Heather Healthcare:

You will recall that Heather had a Calcium score of 0, which is the best score possible. It means she has no signs of heart disease, and doesn't have to worry about that for about 10 years. But Healther was interested in the "Top of Calling" added functionality. She continues to work as a nurse in traditional medicine, but has also started counseling sessions with heart disease patients. Heather undergoes subsequent screenings at 10-year intervals (ages 45, 55, etc.). While minor changes may occur, her scores remain low, indicating she maintains her preventative focus. Heather lives a long, healthy life, largely free of cardiac events. She benefits from continuous, proactive, preventative care guided by her initial zero score. Heather lived until the age of 91.

The Heather Healthcare persona is intended to help us understand the point of view of the caregiver role within the Elevate Health community. She represents the family members, friends, or professional aides who need limited care and primarily provide care and support to patients. The caregiver role is one of the most critical roles of the Elevate Health Community. These individuals are motivated by a singular purpose: to ensure their loved one receives the best possible care. Their needs, therefore, are centered on finding reliable information, having intuitive tools to manage appointments and medications, and coordinating with a diverse cast of healthcare providers.

Caregivers often play a critical role in decision-making, logistics, and emotional support. It's the caregiver who frequently must bridge between the patient's needs and the complexities of the healthcare system. This is a complicated and thankless task. It grinds our caregivers down every day in the traditional healthcare industry. The caregiver role demands support tools providing efficient communication and resources to manage overhead. Many of the early utilities in the Elevate Health market will be to help caregivers. Without these tools, they are left to navigate a labyrinth of paperwork and phone calls, all while juggling the emotional and physical demands of caring for their father, patient, or member.

This relentless pressure highlights the significant challenges caregivers face daily. They are at a high risk of burnout, often lacking adequate support networks and experiencing immense stress from the constant demands of care coordination. A key frustration is the difficulty in accessing patient information, often hindered by privacy regulations or fragmented healthcare systems. These challenges underscore a critical opportunity in the Elevate Health 2050 market. By recognizing and actively supporting the caregiver's vital role, we can create a system that provides intuitive tools for communication, streamlined coordination, and easy access to support networks. Ultimately, these caregivers will be able to step up and serve as a primary positive influence on a Member's goals, outlook, and ultimately the utilization of the Elevate Health system.

Andy Armstrong

Andy was interested in learning about the Heart Health program, but is primarily interested in exploring a business opportunity for his company. He had a Calcium score of 5, indicating the beginning of heart disease. Andy was intrigued by the AI-Coach and learned all about heart disease and his options. He discussed the results with his primary care doctor and began taking a daily Statin. Andy chats with the AI-Coach over the years, getting personalized dietary advice and help with stress management. He successfully manages his cardiac risk and adds remote monitoring in his later years to help him stabilize and manage his heart disease. While his business involves significant stress, the proactive management offsets much of the risk. Andy successfully avoids a premature heart attack but experiences general wear and tear related to his high-stress career and initial low risk. His engagement with Elevate Health's services helps him live a full and healthy life until his death at age 79.

The Andy Armstrong persona represents the builders, entrepreneurs, developers, service providers, and business leaders who create new solutions and build the Elevate Health market. Andy's trajectory demonstrates the effectiveness of the system for individuals with minimal detectable risk who actively engage in intervention. Andy's score of 5 triggers the triage system, since even a low-positive Calcium score indicates the presence of heart disease. Despite being relatively young, the system identifies Andy as needing intervention. Andy, being a CEO focused on efficiency and outcomes, recognizes the value of the intervention. He engages with the market's specialized programs to manage his risk.

Builders, like Andy, are catalysts for change. They are motivated by identifying inefficiencies and gaps in the existing market. Andy wants to create scalable solutions that deliver value, whether through technology, specialized services, or new operational models. Builders face significant hurdles, including navigating complex regulatory environments, securing partnerships with established institutions, obtaining funding, and integrating new technologies with existing legacy systems. They are looking for clear pathways to integrate their services, secure funding, and achieve positive outcomes for patients and their own profits. Andy is motivated by the potential for high impact and market disruption.

Paul Patient

Unlike Andy and Heather, Paul is an example of a noncompliant patient. You will recall that Paul only grudgingly went to the Heart Health Calcium Screen at his wife's request. His Calcium score was 75, indicating significant heart disease. Unfortunately, Paul elected to ignore his health issues and took no action. He is unmotivated and slightly paralyzed by fear. The AI-Coach remains available to him, but it cannot mandate Member engagement. Paul resists any further testing or health interventions. He dismisses the risk because he doesn't have any negative symptoms and finds the suggested lifestyle changes too disruptive. Without intervention, Paul's heart disease progresses unchecked. The calcification worsens over the next two decades, leading to advanced coronary artery disease. The cumulative effects of his sedentary lifestyle and refusal to engage with the preventative measures led to a sudden, fatal cardiac event. Sadly, Paul at the young age of 58.

The Paul Patient persona represents the unmotivated population. Unfortunately, this group represents a significant percentage of the overall population. Elevate Health strives to educate members to help them understand that they have many tools to improve and enhance their health and overall quality of life. Yet, if a patient is not engaged and unmotivated to improve their health, our community grants them the freedom to chart their own path. Paul highlights that while the infrastructure enables opportunity, individual agency remains key to health and wellness. The infrastructure and capabilities are in place, but not all individuals will engage.

Ellie Engagement

Ellie learned about the Heart Health Calcium Screening from her sister and went because it was free and convenient. However, when Ellie gets her Calcium score result of 75, she leans in and engages with the Elevate health system. Ellie is motivated by the results of her screening. She is pragmatic and understands the gravity of the elevated score, choosing to trust the AI-Coach's guidance. Ellie finds a Cardiologist through the Elevate Health Community and begins to focus on improving her health. She is prescribed daily Statin medication, begins doing yoga 3 times per week, and sets a goal to begin eating a healthier diet. Over time, the Elevate Health Market provides Ellie with access to specialized programs and dedicated caregiver support. She is able to manage her heart disease and live longer because the infrastructure supports her active participation. Ellie successfully avoids a premature heart attack, and her engagement with Elevate Health's services helps her live a full and healthy life until her death at 79 years of age.

Ellie represents a Member with significant underlying risk who chooses to engage with the Elevate Health Market. Unlike Paul, who resists the diagnosis, Ellie is motivated by the objective data from her screening. She is pragmatic and understands the gravity of the elevated score, choosing to trust the market's guidance. Upon receiving her score, Ellie is immediately triaged by the AI-Coach and connected to a cardiologist. She accepts the personalized care plan, which includes medications, remote monitoring, enrollment in specialized cardiovascular prevention programs, participation in telehealth consultations, and necessary lifestyle modifications. Through active participation in the Elevate Health Markets, Ellie successfully manages her heart disease.

The comparison between Paul and Ellie is instructive. Paul and Ellie are both successfully screened as having cardiac disease at 35 years of age. However, Paul is disengaged and noncompliant, leading to a premature heart attack at 58 years of age. Ellie has the same initial risk as Paul, but her engagement with the Elevate Health Market's treatments and preventative protocols allows her to live a productive life until 79, matching Andy’s lifespan despite more advanced heart disease at 35. This contrast vividly illustrates one of the core value propositions of the Elevate Health Market: Early detection combined with engaged patients and appropriate intervention can drastically alter the trajectory of cardiac disease and the Member’s life.

Summary

This chapter describes how Elevate Health's innovative market infrastructure is designed to overcome the critical challenges of trust and data control that plague traditional healthcare markets. We achieve this by re-engineering the foundational rules of engagement around our shared values and foundational beliefs. We anticipate leveraging powerful innovations from all three of the innovation waves, with a particular focus on how Web3 technology can facilitate the shared belief in Radical Market Transparency combined with Personal Data Sovereignty. These twin pillars empower individuals by giving them complete control over their health data and allowing them to engage with the market on their own terms. This shift creates a fundamentally more trustworthy and equitable ecosystem. Additionally, the High/Low Margin framework serves as the economic engine, balancing lucrative, high-margin services with essential, low-margin offerings. This strategic approach ensures the ecosystem is self-sufficient and scalable, capable of providing a comprehensive range of services without being solely reliant on external funding or traditional, often inequitable, reimbursement models. This creates a sustainable and equitable healthcare ecosystem designed to thrive in the Intelligence Age.

This robust infrastructure is not merely a short-term fix; it is built to do more than just survive the coming societal crisis. It is a blueprint for thriving in the subsequent "High period," offering a "paint-by-numbers" manual for future leaders to re-imagine and elevate health as a fundamental human right. By establishing a clear, replicable model, Elevate Health provides a tangible path forward for others to follow. The critical infrastructure has been laid, and the foundation is secure. The remaining challenge, which is the focus of subsequent efforts, is to scale the community, inspire broad engagement, and continuously refine the offerings to maximize human quality of life. The framework is ready; the next step is to activate the network and bring this vision to life.

Chapter 7: Builders

It won't mean a thing in 100 years
- Blues Traveler

Everyone is busy in our noisy, always-on world. However, much of our day-to-day activities "won't mean a thing in 100 years." One of the keys to elevating health above politics is a focus on actions and decisions that will impact health markets in the year 2050. In Chapter 4, we discussed Elevate Health's primary purpose: to elevate our attention and effort to our shared health values and foundational beliefs. When we take a wider view and focus on the year 2050, Elevate Health Members believe these values and beliefs will endure. Or at least, we think global human health and wellness will benefit if we can agree on shared values across the entire community. In Chapter 5, we simplified healthcare into the two essential health roles: patient and caregiver. We noted that this interface between the patient and caregiver may be captured by Elevate Health Markets in the form of the Personal Wellness AI-Coach product. We believe that by engaging with the patient or Member, we will learn about them and begin to develop ways to make them healthier. Over many years, this should evolve into a resilient health Market. In this chapter, we turn to the third and final role in creating the Elevate Health Markets: Builders. We do not believe that potential benefits to customers automatically get added to existing systems. In our experience, that is not how innovation occurs. Typically, it is adopted at the edges and then gradually gains acceptance by the overall market. Incumbents often actively resist innovation and change in general. Therefore, markets require an active process of conversion of potential technical capabilities into valuable products.

Builders is the term we use to describe the role of developing new health and wellness products and services. Most people identifying as Builders are focused on long-term impact and strive to create solutions that address the specific needs of individuals. Health builders leave a positive impact on the world by developing and spreading novel health products that create value for patients and caregivers. They go by many names in society today. In some circles, they are called entrepreneurs, founders, product developers or business leaders. All of these roles share many similarities with the Elevate Health concept of Builders. However, these terms also carry embedded assumptions that can cause confusion. We intentionally select the term "Builder" to clearly define the role within Elevate Health Markets.

Builders Defined

Elevate Health Builders creates new consumer surplus through a 4-step process described below. Consumer surplus is an economic concept that quantifies the difference between the highest price a consumer is willing to pay for a good or service and the actual price they pay. This surplus reflects the benefit consumers receive when they purchase a product for less than the maximum they would be willing to pay. For example, if a health consumer wants to lose weight to improve their health and look better, they may assign a value of $1,000/month to this outcome. If they can purchase a GLP1 medication for $600/month, then they have a consumer surplus of $1,000 - $600 = $400 per month. It is the Builders' role to develop and distribute new products and services that increase this surplus. They accomplish this by either creating more than $1,000 in value for the patient or by reducing the cost to less than $600. In this way, Builders are constantly pushing to increase value to consumers while decreasing costs. Markets are highly competitive, and not all attempts at increasing consumer surplus are successful. Over time, some new products are successful and others fail, but the competition drives the market overall to deliver better products to consumers at lower costs.

Four Steps of a Builder

This process of Builders developing new products to increase consumer surplus for patients is as essential to Elevate Health Markets as the relationship between caregivers and patients. There are four critical steps that Builders use to drive positive impact and greater surplus or value for healthcare consumers. Below, we describe each of these steps.

Step 1: Building Empathy

Most people imagine Mark Zuckerberg or Elon Musk as lone inventors who created Facebook or SpaceX and brought them to the world. However, this is not how most builders we work with create products with actual societal impact. Instead, we believe the building process begins by building empathy with a specific customer persona, sometimes referred to as the Ideal Customer Persona, or "ICP," for short. This is a critical part of the process that is often overlooked. In the first stage, Builders invest significant time and energy in deeply understanding their future customers before they move to step 2.

Step 2: Building Insight

The second misconception about Builders is that they intuitively understand the technical capabilities of all available technical innovations. This is not possible in the post-AI environment. The three waves of innovation are propagating much faster than humans can keep up with. No exceptions. However, research is also greatly enhanced by AI. A builder can come up to speed very quickly. Therefore a critical aspect of product development is that builders may not create, nor are they allowed to begin thinking of possible solutions to the ICP's needs and desires, before understanding the solutions making up the status quo. Research is the act of learning what others have done before you in health, biology, AI, software, physics, and psychology. It also includes what the ICP does today to meet these needs and desires, as well as applicable regulations and reimbursement. Importantly, research is NOT idea generation. We know AI systems will tell Builders how brilliant they are. Resist. While it is an ego boost to try and "invent new physics" in collaboration with a sycompant LLM. This is a waste of time. Research is not ideation.

Once you have unpacked and understood all of the existing Research on technological innovations and established capability. Elevate Health Builders add novelty or "seasoning" in the form of at least three diverse perspectives incorporated and cross-pollinated. This is a critical part of the process because it compels the research to broaden its perspective and view the ICP situation from unique points of view. It drives creativity and novelty in a noisy, vanilla world.

Step 3: Building Ideas

The third part of the process is the classic brainstorming of creative work, which has been taught in design thinking shops for over 25 years. Some builders love this process, while others find it hard to let go of assumptions and break outside standard "industry norms" that limit creativity.

Through the process of building empathy and researching innovation, builders often create entirely new ways to deliver value to the ICP. We refer to this as a value-chain. Often, it will be necessary to consider several links in the overall value chain as more than one may be required for large-scale adoption. We encourage the creation of 300-500 ideas. The goal is to generate numerous ideas without judging any of them as good or bad, or possible or not. Just ideas. These ideas are then added to the research materials in a tagging system, allowing easy collaboration and idea development in the next Product/Market Fit process.

Step 4: Building Impact

The fourth and final part of the process is an iteration between hypothesis, prototype, experiment, results, and updated research/ideation. Builders develop a hypothesis, assemble a few key features, and build a prototype to then show to ICPs and gather their feedback. Initially, builders have poor hypotheses and learn basic lessons from the market. However, as they learn, they can slowly develop better and more detailed hypotheses and begin to learn more valuable and unique lessons. Eventually, they have a product that delivers value in excess of the cost of producing it. This is a version of consumer surplus and what Elevate Health calls a “Member Surplus.”

If builders can increase Members' Surplus, they are likely to have a successful product release. We judge the Product/Market fit to be accomplished when over 50% of the time, the Member representing the ICP market takes the prototype and begins using it for the intended purpose. This may be at a free or premium level. They do not have to pay. It is hard enough to achieve 50% usage. Only after the product is “fit to the market” do we turn to develop product pricing and other aspects of the business model to enable delivery of the product to many members. The iterative process of product refinement continues even once Product/Market fit is achieved. Builders must walk a fine line between constantly iterating and improving product and sales, deployment and scaling market adoption.

Builders within the Elevate Health Market:

As discussed in previous chapters, Builders in Elevate Health Markets leverage the values, beliefs, and overall market infrastructure. The goal of a healthy healthcare ecosystem is not to eliminate profits but to align incentives so that all organizations are working toward the same objective: improving health for all. The traditional division between for-profit and non-profit healthcare organizations is a false choice that misrepresents the reality of a functional market. Every organization, regardless of its tax status, must generate sufficient revenue to cover its operational costs, including personnel, equipment, and facilities. We propose replacing the for-profit/non-profit binary choice with a more transparent, two-tiered system: High-Margin and Low-Margin organizations. This approach ensures financial sustainability and creates a self-sustaining ecosystem where innovation fuels accessibility.

Building Public Health Utilities:

The foundation of the Elevate Health Market structure is the Low-Margin organization. We are looking for Builders to help create the "public health utilities" of the future, responsible for delivering essential, established public health, wellness, diagnostic, and preventative services. By design, these organizations maintain a gross margin of under 15%, ensuring that their services remain affordable and accessible to the entire community. Often leveraging established healthcare best practices and well-documented science, these entities are critical for addressing widespread health challenges and ensuring that basic care is not a luxury. Builders will use these organizations for labor-intensive healthcare services or to deliver valuable open-source intellectual property. These organizations provide the fundamental services that improve population health outcomes and form the bedrock of a strong health market. In Chapter 9, we will be illustrating this process by describing the building of a Remote Patient Monitoring public utility product for the Ellie persona.

Building Health Innovations:

Many Builders will also be interested in developing products at the other end of the spectrum using Elevate Health's High-Margin organizations. These are the "innovation drivers" that develop new and transformative methods for diagnosing, treating, and managing health issues. They attract top talent and capital by offering the potential for significant returns, and as a result, they can push the boundaries of medical science and technology. To ensure these High-Margin organizations contribute to the common good, they are required to contribute 10% of their revenues back to the community in the form of free services, educational content, or direct financial contributions. This creates a powerful and positive flywheel: the more these innovative companies earn, the more they are required to invest in free or Low-Margin utilities, directly funding the infrastructure that makes public health services widely available.

This two-category framework also creates clear pathways for accessing capital. High-Margin organizations, with their focus on growth and profitability, are a natural fit for equity markets, including venture capital, private equity, and public stock offerings. This access to capital allows them to scale rapidly and fund ambitious research and development projects. Conversely, Low-Margin organizations are better suited for debt and bond markets, which provide the stable, long-term financing needed to maintain their essential, utility-like functions. By aligning an organization's margin profile with the appropriate capital source,

Builders are able to seek the proper capital partners, ensuring a more stable and efficient market.

Builders who develop a deep understanding of human needs are best positioned for success within the Elevate Health ecosystem. Their four-step process—building Empathy, Insight, Ideas, and Impact—naturally aligns with the needs of members. Builders offer their products and services directly to members through the interface of a Personal Wellness AI-Coach, creating a mutually beneficial relationship. For their products to be successful, they must be designed to increase "Member's Surplus," meaning they provide a value that exceeds their cost, and offer a positive, member-centric experience. This model creates a useful balance of power. While builders are motivated by profit, the entire system is fundamentally designed to optimize for the member's health and wellness, ensuring that the market's primary focus remains on improving individual well-being rather than commercial gain.

This symbiotic relationship fuels growth. Builders, whether operating with low or high margins, strive to innovate and increase the value they provide to members. As they succeed, they earn profits that can be reinvested into their organizations, allowing them to develop their ideas further and expand their offerings. This cycle of innovation and reinvestment creates a dynamic market where new tools, services, and technologies are constantly being introduced to better serve member needs. This growth is not explosive or chaotic; instead, it's a slow and steady process that protects the independence and long-term resilience of the Elevate Health ecosystem.

By prioritizing deliberate, sustainable growth over rapid expansion, the Elevate Health Market protects its core principles. This approach ensures that the ecosystem remains resilient and independent from external pressures, such as venture capital or corporate interests, that might prioritize profit over member health. This model enables the organization to remain agile and faithful to its mission of empowering members to take control of their health. It’s the difference between a tree with deep roots that can weather any storm and a fast-growing weed that is easily pulled from the ground. This model also makes Elevate Health exceptionally scalable and resilient, making it well-suited for navigating future crises. In times of economic hardship, when individuals may lose their traditional healthcare coverage, the market can quickly expand to support them. The decentralized, member-centric structure allows for rapid adaptation and deployment of new solutions, ensuring that essential health services remain accessible. This adaptability positions the Elevate Health Market not only to survive but to thrive, emerging as a leading health market by 2050 by proving its ability to provide consistent, high-quality care, regardless of external circumstances.

Andy Armstrong becomes a Builder:

Let's explore how our Key Persona - Andy Armstrong builds a new wellness product. This helps ground the abstract policy discussion to the actual people innovating in healthcare. You will recall that we first met the Andy persona in Chapter 4. He represents the builders, entrepreneurs, developers, service providers, and business leaders who create new solutions and build products within the Elevate Health market. Andy's Calcium score of 5 triggers the triage system, since even a low-positive score indicates the presence of heart disease. Despite being relatively young, the system identifies Andy as needing intervention. Andy, being a CEO focused on efficiency and outcomes, recognizes the value of the intervention. He engages with the market's specialized programs to manage his personal health risks.

However, Andy is also a builder and is motivated by the potential for high impact and the goal of helping others improve their health. He is motivated by identifying inefficiencies and gaps in the existing market. Andy wants to create scalable solutions that deliver value or as we now refer to it, increased Member Surplus. Andy is attracted to the idea of leveraging AI tools and the Clean-room Reverse Engineering process to develop a new and more affordable GLP-1 type medication.

Andy's Builds Empathy (step #1)

He first builds empathy with the specific Ideal Customer Persona (ICP) that he wants to help. For Andy's case, he wants to help patients who are both overweight and have at least one chronic disease. He interviews 30 members who fit this ICP, asking open-ended questions to learn as much as possible and truly empathize with their needs. Through this process, Andy learns that his target ICP gives a high value to the benefits of the GLP-1 medication. However, they are also very worried about the high cost and fearful that they will not be able to afford the important medication for long. In addition, about 50% of the interviewees are unhappy with the stomach issues that these drugs have as side effects. Andy believes that he can use the clean-room reverse engineering IP process to develop less expensive GLP-1-like medications. He is uncertain about the possibility of reducing the adverse side effects, but plans to investigate further.

Andy Builds Insight (step #2)

Andy then turns to researching the GLP-1 Market to gain insight into the status quo products. He learns that the Glucagon-like peptide-1 (GLP-1) receptor agonists represent one of the most significant pharmaceutical breakthroughs of the 21st century. These compounds were first approved for the treatment of type 2 diabetes in 2005. Since this time, these drugs have revolutionized treatment approaches for both diabetes and obesity, with recent approvals expanding their indications significantly. The clinical significance of GLP-1 receptor agonists cannot be overstated. These drugs work by mimicking the action of the naturally occurring hormone GLP-1, which helps regulate blood sugar levels and slows gastric emptying, leading to improved glycemic control and significant weight loss. The most prominent examples include:

- Semaglutide (Ozempic, Wegovy, Rybelsus): Developed by Novo Nordisk
- Liraglutide (Victoza, Saxenda): Developed by Novo Nordisk
- Dulaglutide (Trulicity): Developed by Eli Lilly
- Exenatide (Byetta, Bydureon): Developed by Amylin Pharmaceuticals

The market for these drugs has experienced significant growth in recent years, with global sales now exceeding tens of billions of dollars annually. However, their high cost has created significant access barriers, with monthly treatment costs often exceeding $1,000 per patient.

We selected this market opportunity because the intellectual property landscape surrounding GLP-1 receptor agonists is extraordinarily complex and strategically constructed to maximize market exclusivity for incumbents. Andy finds research published in JAMA revealing the sophisticated patent strategies employed by pharmaceutical manufacturers. Multinational pharmaceutical companies have created robust IP protection, with an average of 19.5 patents per GLP-1 receptor agonist. This has created a "dense thicket" of patents that pose significant barriers to entry by others - including Andy. These patents cover multiple aspects of the drugs:

- Active Ingredient Patents: Covering the specific peptide sequences and their modifications
- Formulation Patents: Protecting specific pharmaceutical compositions and excipients
- Delivery Device Patents: Covering injection pens, auto-injectors, and other delivery mechanisms
- Method of Use Patents: Protecting specific therapeutic applications and dosing regimens
- Manufacturing Process Patents: Covering production methods and purification techniques

Additionally, these companies have been able to extend the effective IP protection significantly longer than the standard 20-year patent term from the 2005 initial filing. This extension is achieved through: filing continuation patents and improvements over time, combining drug patents with delivery and device patents, and developing new formulations that extend patent life. The complexity of the GLP-1 patent landscape has created formidable barriers to generic competition. Andy notes in his research, "No generic firm has successfully challenged patents on GLP-1 receptor agonists to gain FDA approval."

Andy Builds Ideas (step #3)

Andy explores multiple ideas but lands on one to develop further. He names the Project "Metabolic Freedom" to symbolize the unlocking of the GLP-1 Technology for large numbers of Members that are overweight and suffering from a chronic disease related to metabolic dysregulation, including Diabetes, Cardiovascular Disease, and Kidney Disease, among others. This project represents a hypothetical but technically feasible application of AI-assisted clean room methodology to develop a novel GLP-1 receptor agonist.

Andy also identifies an AI tool called Evo2 to help him in developing Project Metabolic Freedom. Evo2 is a groundbreaking biological foundation AI model capable of predicting and designing DNA sequences across various organisms, including humans, animals, plants, and microbes. It was developed by scientists at

Arc Institute in collaboration with NVIDIA and researchers from Stanford University, UC Berkeley, and UC San Francisco. Andy seeks to combine the power of Evo2's genomic AI capabilities and rigorous clean room processes to potentially circumvent the extensive patent thickets surrounding existing GLP-1 drugs while creating a superior therapeutic option. His primary goal is to develop a novel GLP-1 receptor agonist that achieves superior therapeutic outcomes compared to existing drugs while avoiding all intellectual property infringement. This will allow him to offer the new medication to Elevate Health members at a far lower price. Secondary objectives include reduction of gastrointestinal side effects, developing novel manufacturing processes, and creating innovative delivery systems.

<u>Andy Builds Impact-Functional Analysis (step #4a)</u>

Andy assembles a team named Team Alpha to develop the functional specifications for the overall project. Team Alpha comprises endocrinologists, pharmacologists, and regulatory experts who have no prior exposure to proprietary information regarding existing GLP-1 drugs. Andy himself does not participate in team Alpha so he does not contaminate himself. Team Alpha members sign comprehensive agreements that prohibit access to proprietary data, patent applications, or confidential information about existing GLP-1 receptor agonists. Team Alpha begins by analyzing the GLP-1 receptor using only publicly available structural data from the Protein Data Bank, published crystallographic studies, and peer-reviewed research papers. They document the receptor's structure, including the seven-transmembrane domain architecture, extracellular binding regions, and intracellular signaling domains. The team identifies the key binding requirements for GLP-1 receptor activation, including the critical amino acid residues involved in ligand recognition, the conformational changes required for G-protein coupling, and the downstream signaling cascades that mediate therapeutic effects. This analysis reveals that for a variety of technical reasons, effective GLP-1 receptor agonists must achieve specific binding affinity thresholds, demonstrate selectivity over related receptors, and produce sustained activation patterns.

Therapeutic Outcome Requirements:

Through analysis of published clinical trial data, medical literature, and FDA regulatory documents,

Team Alpha documents the desired therapeutic profile for an ideal GLP-1 receptor agonist. The specifications include:

- Glycemic control targets of HbA1c reduction of 1.0-1.5% from baseline, fasting glucose reduction of 30-50 mg/dL, and postprandial glucose reduction of 50-80 mg/dL. Weight loss targets of 5-15% body weight reduction over 6-12 months, with sustained weight maintenance over longer periods. Cardiovascular benefits, including reduction in major adverse cardiovascular events, improvement in blood pressure, and favorable lipid profile changes.
- Pharmacokinetic Specifications: The team analyzes published pharmacokinetic data to establish optimal drug exposure profiles. They determine that an ideal GLP-1 receptor agonist should have a half-life of 5-7 days to enable once-weekly dosing, bioavailability of >80% following subcutaneous injection, and minimal drug-drug interactions through non-CYP metabolic pathways.
- Safety Profile Requirements: Through comprehensive analysis of safety data from

published studies and regulatory documents, Team Alpha establishes the safety specifications for the novel compound. These include minimization of gastrointestinal side effects, absence of pancreatitis risk, no increased risk of thyroid C-cell tumors, and compatibility with common diabetes medications.

Andy Builds Impact- Design (step #4b)

Evo2 represents a groundbreaking advancement in biological foundation models, developed by the Arc Institute and released in early 2025. This genomic foundation model is capable of generalist prediction and design tasks across DNA, RNA, and proteins, utilizing a frontier deep learning architecture that enables modeling of biological sequences at single-nucleotide resolution with near-linear scaling of compute and memory relative to context length. The model's specifications are unprecedented in the field of computational biology:

- Scale: Trained with 40 billion parameters on over 9.3 trillion nucleotides of diverse eukaryotic and prokaryotic genomes
- Context Window: 1 megabase context length, allowing analysis of entire genomic regions

- Resolution: Single-nucleotide resolution for precise genetic analysis
- Scope: Spans all domains of life, from prokaryotes to complex eukaryotic organisms
- Capabilities: Both predictive analysis and generative design of biological sequences

Evo2's capabilities extend far beyond traditional sequence analysis tools. The model demonstrates remarkable proficiency in accurately predicting the functional impacts of genetic variation. This capability suggests the model has learned some fundamental principles of how genetic sequences translate to biological function. Furthermore, researchers have announced that Evo2 autonomously learns a breadth of biological features, including exon-intron boundaries, transcription factor binding sites, protein structural elements, and prophage genomic regions. This suggests the model has developed an internal representation of biological complexity that mirrors our best collective scientific understanding.

The Evo2 system is configured with access only to the functional specifications developed by Team Alpha, publicly available genomic databases, and fundamental biological principles. The AI system has no access to proprietary information about existing GLP-1 drugs, patent databases, or confidential pharmaceutical data. Evo2 analyzes the GLP-1 receptor structure and functional requirements to generate novel peptide sequences that could achieve optimal receptor activation. The AI leverages its understanding of protein-protein interactions, learned from its training on billions of genomic sequences, to predict peptide sequences that would bind effectively to the GLP-1 receptor. Andy and the AI collaborate to generate multiple candidate sequences, each designed to meet specific aspects of the functional requirements. Some candidates are optimized for binding affinity, others for selectivity, and still others for stability and pharmacokinetic properties. The AI's analysis reveals that certain amino acid modifications could potentially enhance the properties of the natural GLP-1 hormone.

Evo2 generates a series of novel peptide sequences that incorporate non-natural amino acids, modified peptide bonds, and innovative structural features designed to enhance therapeutic properties. One up-and-coming candidate, designated "EvoGLP-1α," incorporates several novel features: A modified N-terminus that enhances receptor binding affinity through additional hydrogen bonding interactions. Strategic incorporation of D-amino acids to improve proteolytic stability without compromising biological activity. A novel C-terminal extension that facilitates albumin binding for extended half-life. Cyclization through a disulfide bridge that stabilizes the active conformation.

Andy works with the AI system to analyze the generated sequences for predicted pharmacokinetic properties, using its understanding of protein structure-function relationships to optimize absorption, distribution, and clearance characteristics. Evo2 predicts that EvoGLP-1α would have a half-life of approximately 6 days, excellent subcutaneous bioavailability, and minimal immunogenicity risk. Leveraging its ability to predict functional impacts of sequence variations, Evo2 analyzes the generated compounds for potential safety issues. The AI predicts that EvoGLP-1α would have reduced gastrointestinal side effects compared to existing drugs due to its modified receptor activation profile, while maintaining full therapeutic efficacy.

Andy Builds Impact- Product Sythesis (step #4c):

Next, Andy needs to build his "clean" human team. He names this team Beta, and it consists of medicinal chemists, formulation scientists, and manufacturing experts. None of these team Beta members has any knowledge of Team Alpha's analysis process or existing GLP-1 drugs. They receive only the AI-generated specifications and functional requirements, without any information on how these specifications were derived. Team Beta synthesizes EvoGLP-1α using standard solid-phase peptide synthesis techniques, incorporating the novel structural features specified by the AI system. Initial characterization confirms the predicted molecular weight, purity, and structural integrity of the compound. Biological activity testing reveals that EvoGLP-1α demonstrates superior GLP-1 receptor binding affinity compared to the natural hormone, with an IC50 of 0.8 nM compared to 5.2 nM for native GLP-1. The compound shows excellent selectivity over related receptors and produces sustained cAMP elevation in target cells.

The team also develops a novel subcutaneous injection formulation for EvoGLP-1α, incorporating innovative excipients and stabilizers to maintain peptide integrity and optimize injection comfort. The formulation includes a novel buffer system that maintains an optimal pH and prevents aggregation. Proprietary stabilizers that protect against oxidation and deamidation. A co-formulated local anesthetic to minimize injection site discomfort. An innovative delivery system that enables precise dosing and improved patient compliance. Team Beta develops a completely novel manufacturing process for EvoGLP-1α that incorporates several innovative elements, including a proprietary cell-free synthesis system that eliminates the need for bacterial or mammalian cell culture. Novel purification techniques that achieve >99% purity with minimal processing steps. Innovative lyophilization processes that maintain peptide stability during storage. Quality control systems that ensure batch-to-batch consistency and regulatory compliance.

The team conducts comprehensive preclinical studies demonstrating EvoGLP-1α's superior therapeutic profile. In diabetic animal models, the compound achieves better glycemic control than existing drugs while producing greater weight loss and fewer side effects. Toxicology studies reveal an excellent safety profile with no concerning findings.

Andy Builds Impact- Regulation (step #4d):

Andy works with team Beta to design an innovative clinical trial that can demonstrate EvoGLP-1α's superior therapeutic profile, based solely on the functional specifications and preclinical results. The trials incorporate novel endpoints and patient populations that highlight the compound's unique advantages. Phase I studies focus on safety, tolerability, and pharmacokinetics in healthy volunteers and patients with type 2 diabetes. The studies reveal that EvoGLP-1α has a half-life of 6.2 days, enabling true once-weekly dosing, and produces dose-proportional increases in drug exposure. Phase II studies demonstrate superior efficacy compared to historical controls, with HbA1c reductions of 1.4% and a 12% weight loss over 26 weeks. Notably, the studies show significantly reduced gastrointestinal side effects, with only 8% of patients experiencing nausea compared to typical rates of 20-40% with existing drugs. The development team collaborates with regulatory authorities to establish novel approval pathways that recognize the innovative features of EvoGLP-1α. The compound receives breakthrough therapy designation based on its superior efficacy and safety profile, enabling accelerated development timelines.

Andy Builds Impact- Intellectual Property (step #4e):

Throughout the development process, comprehensive patent applications are filed covering EvoGLP-1α's novel sequence, formulation, manufacturing processes, and clinical applications. The patent strategy focuses on creating strong, defensible intellectual property that protects the innovations developed through the clean room process. However, Andy plans to make this IP available to any Low-Margin Organizations after 3 years in alignment with the Elevate Health Market practices. He also plans to sell the drug at high margins and reinvest 10% of revenue into free educational services.

Andy Builds Impact Analysis (step #4f)

This product has benefits relative to the existing GLP-1 medications, and it is also has significant cost advantages. The innovative manufacturing approach reduces production costs by approximately 60%, while the improved efficacy and reduced side effects enhance overall cost-effectiveness. Economic modeling suggests that EvoGLP-1α could be priced at 40-50% below existing GLP-1 drugs while maintaining attractive profit margins. This pricing strategy would dramatically improve patient access while generating substantial revenue for the developing company.

Andy Launches the Product

Andy introduces EvoGLP-1α, which represents a significant market disruption by cutting the price point to $200/month and capturing substantial market share from existing drugs through superior clinical outcomes and improved affordability. The compound's novel features could establish new treatment paradigms and expand the overall GLP-1 market. The success of Project "Metabolic Freedom" prompts competitive responses from existing pharmaceutical companies, accelerating innovation in the GLP-1 space and ultimately benefiting patients through improved therapeutic options and increased competition.

Legal and Ethical Considerations

This example is fictional, but plausible. Elevate Health expects this AI-assisted clean-room process to negatively impact pharmaceutical companies and all organizations relying on an IP portfolio. IP is no longer broadly enforceable as anyone can reverse engineer the IP in a relatively short amount of time in collaboration with the waves of innovation from AI, Web3, and Biotech. It seems likely that there will be hundreds of Andy-like Builders in the next several years. However, Elevate Health's vision is that the commoditization of Intelligence can be powerful for the overall community of open-source projects. We can channel a lot of power, influence, and capital by bringing these innovations to benefit everyone. Often, these will be excellent candidates to become low-margin health utilities in the Elevate Health market.

The clean room methodology employed in Project "Metabolic Freedom" provides strong legal protection against intellectual property infringement claims. The rigorous separation between analysis and implementation teams, combined with comprehensive documentation of the development process, creates a robust defense against allegations of patent infringement. The use of AI systems like Evo2 adds a layer of protection, as the AI's analysis is based on fundamental biological principles rather than reverse engineering of existing compounds. The AI's ability to generate novel solutions from functional requirements provides strong evidence of independent creation. This example raises essential questions about the regulatory and ethical framework for AI-generated pharmaceuticals. Regulatory authorities will need to develop new guidelines for evaluating AI-generated compounds and ensuring their safety and efficacy. The ethical implications of using AI to circumvent pharmaceutical patents also require careful consideration. While the clean room methodology is legally sound, it challenges the traditional pharmaceutical business model and could have significant implications for innovation incentives and drug pricing.

Future Implications for the Pharmaceutical Industry

The success of AI-assisted clean room pharmaceutical development could fundamentally transform the pharmaceutical industry. The question is when these types of new product development processes are possible, not if. This timing uncertainty is one of the primary reasons Elevate Health elected to focus on 2050. The 25-year time horizon is sufficiently out in the future that these types of reverse-engineered products will be viable. Whenever it occurs, the democratization of drug development capabilities through AI tools like Evo2 could enable smaller companies and academic institutions to compete with large pharmaceutical corporations. This transformation could lead to increased competition, lower drug prices, and accelerated innovation. However, it could also disrupt existing business models and potentially reduce incentives for pharmaceutical research and development investment. This illustration of a new product disrupting the GLP-1 market, while fictional, is plausible today. Existing technology is sufficient to enable this type of clean room methodology today with minimal time and resources. This is why the Elevate Health community must develop a new policy quickly. We want to encourage and incentivize both Humans and AIs to invest capital and time in researching to invent or discover new forms of intelligence. How can we create these incentives in the Intelligence Age? The key is to use our shared Values and Beliefs to develop an IP policy that benefits the community as a whole and can be easily enforced.

What Do We Tell: Louisa?

When we consider the future leader we are writing this health market policy book for, we don't imagine the President of the US. While our community would love to be able to serve our country in any way, the US may not need our help. While it is true that the coming crisis could end badly with a Chinese or other non-US leader, we prefer not to dwell on that scenario. Instead, we have a more motivating future Member within the Elevate Health Community.

We imagine a brilliant and hardworking, yet poor, Latina mother of three: Louisa. She is the leader of the non-profit group of families with kids diagnosed with a rare genetic disease. Often, they lose insurance coverage, and many of these kids live outside of their home country and lack the healthcare rights provided to citizens in the state where they live and work. Louisa's group attempts to be transparent about the difficulty in establishing a new and independent healthcare system. Louisa needs the experienced Builders in the Elevate Health community to help her find a way to provide healthcare for her group's kids. Yet we also must be honest about how hard it is to change the status quo in healthcare. Louisa needs to understand the challenges well enough to develop successful strategies to unlock Member Surplus for herself and her community. Elevate Health strives to be prepared to welcome groups of people in need who seek basic health and wellness services. This gives them the opportunity to refuse and allows them to consider becoming a Caregiver or Builder.

Market Layer Cake Analogy:

Delphi Digital is one of the leading research and investment firms in the Web3 space. They have conducted some interesting research on market infrastructure, new product development, and community reinvestment. They have lots of great work, but we have adopted their concept of a layer cake as an analogy to help describe how an overall market functions in a self-sustaining way over time.

Delphi is best known for this "layer cake" framework, a model they pioneered in Web3 to categorize and analyze market opportunities. This structured approach enables Delphi to systematically identify the areas with the most significant potential within a complex ecosystem, ranging from foundational hardware to consumer-facing applications. By segmenting the market into distinct layers, Delphi can more effectively assess risks, rewards, and defensible positions, bringing a familiar and proven methodology to a new frontier.

Delphi's AI "layer cake" breaks down the market into five key levels. The Chips Layer forms the base, representing the essential hardware for AI computations. The next level is the Foundation Models Layer, home to the large, general-purpose AI models that underpin many applications. Above that is the Dev Tools and Infrastructure Layer, which provides the essential tools for developers to build and scale applications. Finally, the Application Layer sits at the top, where consumer products are built on the foundations of the other layers. This framework mirrors Delphi's successful approach to Web3, where they provided influential research on everything from Layer 1 blockchains to Layer 2 to DeFi applications. This layered perspective helps Delphi pinpoint opportunities and build conviction.

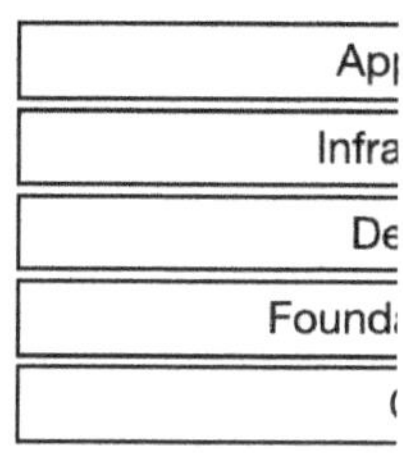
Delphi Digital

Core Principles for Building Community Value

At the Elevate Health Community, we believe that the most successful ventures are built with and for their members. That's why we encourage everyone to get involved in our Builder principles, a set of best practices designed to save time and increase the odds of success for new initiatives. While these principles are not a universal solution, they provide a strong foundation. Every builder should develop their own four-step process—moving from empathy to insight, ideas, and finally, impact. Yet, beyond this foundational process, there are specific principles that can be added to help a product gain significant adoption and lasting impact.

One of the most powerful strategies for creating a sustainable product is aligning the features and Member benefits with the community's values. Once the Builder is aligned with the shared values "layer of the cake," they can offer highly integrated health and wellness coaching, creating significant switching costs. The high switching costs mean health platforms can become so valuable and deeply integrated into a user's life that leaving becomes difficult. This slows adoption without shared values and beliefs. However, once we elevate health through the values, the community fosters far greater trust and member value.

A key element of delivering great experiences and seamless interfaces is the user sharing personal data with the market. By focusing on the values and shared beliefs first, the adoption of data sharing by Elevate Health Members will be faster than in traditional health systems. Similarly, workflow integration is critical. By embedding your product into a user's daily workflow or business processes, you make switching a disruptive and costly endeavor. Beyond that, Builders should strive to offer proprietary features and a superior user experience that competitors cannot easily copy. The power of network effects is extremely powerful in healthcare markets. A network effect occurs when a product's value increases as more users join, just like a social network or a marketplace. In a healthcare community, this means that the more members share knowledge and resources, the more valuable the platform becomes for everyone. This interconnectedness also fosters community trust and reputation, which is paramount in a rapidly evolving and often uncertain space like digital health. A reliable and trustworthy community reduces the perceived risk for users who share sensitive information or adopt new technologies.

Ultimately, these principles work in concert to create a robust and resilient ecosystem. This occurs when the ecosystem begins to add value to all the products. It occurs over time as a platform becomes a central hub by integrating with other essential tools and services—further strengthening its position. By focusing on creating tangible value through unique features, fostering a strong network, and building a trusted community, Elevate Health Builders can develop products that not only attract Members but also retain them as contributing members of the community. This approach transforms a simple health and wellness tool into a valuable part of members' lives in a collaborative community.

Applying the "Layer Cake" to Builders' Principles

Building a successful community-driven platform in the emerging health market requires more than just a great idea; it demands a deliberate strategy for creating both value and stickiness. The Delphi "layer cake" framework provides an excellent model for this, outlining how builders can strategically leverage different technological layers—from applications to infrastructure—to achieve this goal. By integrating AI and Web3 into each layer, innovators in the Elevate Health market can construct a robust, defensible business that not only attracts users but also makes them reluctant to leave.

Win the Application Layer

The most critical layer for building direct community value and switching costs is the Application Layer. This is where members directly interact with the Elevate Health Community, and it's here that deep value can be created. The strategy is to become the undisputed leader for a specific, painful problem within a particular health vertical. Imagine becoming "the AI for Remote Monitoring of Cardiac Disease." The sub-community that forms around this solution becomes synonymous with solving that problem exceptionally well, creating a powerful network effect and a sense of shared purpose that is incredibly difficult to replicate.

The strategic use of AI at the application layer is crucial for building user loyalty. For instance, if an application allows users to continuously input their proprietary data—like personal health records or treatment outcomes—it uses AI to create a deeply personalized knowledge base. Switching to another platform would mean rebuilding this entire knowledge base from scratch, a significant switching cost. Furthermore, users invest time in customizing the AI's behavior, personality, and output style, making this "trained AI" an invaluable asset that is unique to them, as captured by Delphi's "an app for you" concept. Integrating the AI application directly into existing healthcare workflows and focusing on a delightful user experience also makes the solution indispensable. Since a truly elegant and intuitive health AI interface has yet to emerge, the builder who can define this experience will capture significant market share.

Web3 technologies add another powerful dimension to building value at the application layer. The concept of decentralized data ownership, where users truly own their health data on a secure ledger, empowers them. While they can revoke access at any time, the convenience of having their data seamlessly integrated with a superior AI application creates a strong pull factor. Think of it as a form of a personalized vault. Additionally, token-based loyalty and rewards programs can offer tangible, accumulating benefits like discounts or governance rights, further incentivizing continued engagement. For unique or valuable AI outputs, such as personalized care plans or research insights, using NFTs or blockchain records to prove authenticity and ownership can add a layer of verifiable value and stickiness.

Leverage the Infrastructure Layer

At the Infrastructure Layer, value and switching costs can be built through the underlying technological foundations. Leveraging decentralized compute or storage networks, for example, offers developers cost efficiencies, censorship resistance, and uptime guarantees that centralized alternatives may lack. This provides a compelling value proposition that acts as a form of switching cost. Facilitating shared, decentralized training of AI models allows developers to contribute resources and gain ownership of the resulting models, creating a vested interest in the platform's success. Furthermore, integrating on-chain governance will enable developers to have a say in the platform's evolution, fostering a more deeper sense of commitment and community ownership.

Explore the Developer Tools Layer

While the developer-facing Dev Tools Layer may seem less direct, it's a vital part of the "layer cake" for building a sticky ecosystem. The goal here is to dominate developer mindshare. By becoming the "go-to" toolkit for building specific types of AI applications, a company can create powerful switching costs. If your tools require a specialized skill set or become the industry standard, developers will naturally be less likely to switch. A rich ecosystem of compatible libraries, plugins, and a vibrant developer community also fosters loyalty. By offering unique features and superior performance, such as faster model inference or better security, a platform can solidify its position and make it difficult for competitors to catch up.

Outsource Foundational Model and Chips Layers

Finally, at the Foundational Model and Chips layers, where capital intensity is high, Elevate Health Builders should focus on fostering broad access and strategic partnerships, effectively outsourcing these needs rather than building models from scratch. The strategy is to be recognized for having a comprehensive Developer, Infrastructure, and Application ecosystem, and then to foster easy "plug and play" access to a wide range of diverse models. Web3 tools can be used to offer decentralized model inference networks to provide Elevate Health members access to a range of frontier large language models (LLMs), offering resilience and censorship resistance crucial for sensitive healthcare data. Additionally, token-gated access to premium models can create a vested interest, and using blockchain to verify the origin and integrity of AI outputs is critical in sensitive health markets. These strategies ensure that Elevate Health Builders have the freedom to operate and build whatever health and wellness products they want to test out on whatever chip and underlying model is best suited for the task..

Conclusion

The convergence of the three waves of Innovation presents unprecedented opportunities for value creation. Elevate Health expects these potential benefits through a 4-step process to Build: Empathy,

Insight, Ideas, and Impact. This process is how potential or theoretical value is converted to real Member Surplus, benefiting all market participants. The chapter provided a fictional illustration of the clean-room reverse engineering process. It also laid out significant details to help future Builders.

Chapter 8: Public Health for the People

Health is one of the fundamental rights of every human being without distinction of race, religion, political belief, economic or social condition.

- *World Health Organization Constitution, 1946*

The first of Elevate Health's values is that Health is a Human Right. This is the most foundational aspect of our community. If you are human, we believe that you hold a sovereign right to your health identity, health data, and health rights. We also believe that this right should be funded and guaranteed by the communities, states, and religious organizations with which you identify. Unfortunately, this is not the reality many people live in today. Migration of humans out of less developed communities, states, and religious organizations has caused significant increases in both "legal" and "illegal" immigrants over the last 20 years. This has led to a checkerboard of health rights and funded services across the globe, serving as an outward sign that the current world order is beginning to fracture. For simplicity's sake, we illustrate the challenges with the policies of the United States Department of Health and Human Services. These policies differ in other regions of the world, but the general concepts remain the same.

Typically, countries like the US offer a foundational health benefit funding source to reimburse communities, states, and healthcare organizations in delivering care to their population. In the US, this is called Medicaid. The US Government, through Health and Human Services (HHS), provides funding for the health treatment of the poorest US adult citizens and legal immigrants. Medicaid also funds the treatment of 100% of children physically located in the US. However, there are millions of “illegal” or “undocumented” immigrants living, working, and having babies in the US today.

We observe the tension in translating this Federal Policy into State administrative services and implementation of health services (funded by HHS). The different approaches became apparent as the Trump administration changed federal Medicaid policy to require proof of work for all recipients. Prior to these changes, in liberal states like California and my birth state of Massachusetts, ALL humans were included and funded, without anyone looking at or worrying about the human's legal status or citizenship cards. Unfortunately, these states now have the difficult duty of removing millions of undocumented immigrants from the healthcare systems that have been treating them for years. This will be difficult to accomplish and very unpopular with the population. The result will be unhappy people and an increase in uncompensated care within the healthcare systems of these states. In conservative states like Texas and my current home state of Tennessee, patients have always been required to have clear documentation of either US citizenship or permanent visa residency. Only healthcare treatments of humans with these documents have been funded by Medicaid. In these states, the undocumented population does not receive much in health services from the state and local governments. Yet in the wake of the Trump changes to Medicaid, this complete lack of governmental funding actually resulted in other organizations with diverse funding sources attempting to deliver healthcare services. These groups do great work in challenging circumstances, but they often lack sufficient funding to implement best practices in complex clinical healthcare.

Elevate Health attempts to remain agnostic to these political debates. We do not enter into a discussion of the relative pros or cons of either the liberal or conservative approaches. This is not our place. Our goal is to elevate public health above petty political squabbles and establish health rights for individuals. Over time, these shared values and beliefs will evolve into an elevated health market. The hope is that many communities, states, and religious organizations will elect to outsource their health policy, values, and services to the Elevate Health Community.

1st Member Benefit: Foundations

The first Elevate Health Member benefit provides a set of basic human health rights and services, 100% free of charge and hassle-free. If you are human, you may become a Member of Elevate Health and then immediately receive any of the health services included in the Elevate Health Market. Today, as we are just getting started, the community offers few services. In Chapter 10, we will explore growing the market capabilities. These aspirations can be framed as "increasing the ceiling" of the best health treatments for specific types of Members. However, our public health efforts are focused on "raising the floor" for the entire global population of 10 billion people by the year 2050. To ensure access for all, this core set of tools and services, named "Foundations," is provided free to all Elevate Health Members. Foundations provides Members with the best available: health identity, health data, and health rights. It represents Elevate Health's public health offerings, built for the people and funded by the communities, states, and religious organizations to which they belong.

As we described in Chapter 3, the last High Period or Turning in Neil Howe's nomenclature, following the end of World War II, saw the creation of new international organizations designed to address global challenges with coordinated action. The most significant of these related to health was the World Health Organization (WHO). It was designed to coordinate global health efforts through a centralized organizational structure. The first World Health Assembly, held in 1948, included representatives from 53 states from across the world. This assembly established the precedent for global decision-making on health issues and created the institutional framework that would enable coordinated international health initiatives. One of the most important actions was the formal codification of health as a human right. WHO adopted the Universal Declaration of Human Rights within the preamble to its Constitution. The document reads as follows:

> *WHO Constitution:*
> *The enjoyment of the highest attainable standard of health is one of the fundamental rights of every human being without distinction of race, religion, political belief, economic or social condition.*

This was the first time that the right to health was formally recognized in an international legal document. The WHO constitution further established a broad definition of health, which it defined as "a state of complete physical, mental, and social well-being and not merely the absence of disease or infirmity."

Public Health during the 3 Waves

Public health is the science of protecting and improving the health of people and entire communities. In the next 25 years, the 3 waves of innovation AI, Web3, and Biotech will dramatically improve the effectiveness of healthcare services. These improvements will be one or two orders of magnitude more powerful. This means that our technology tools will get 10x to 100x more powerful. It can be challenging to fully comprehend the impact of a two orders of magnitude change in technical capability. Suffice it to say, the potential for unlocking more Member Surplus far exceeds what Builders can convert into valuable products and services.

However, there will also be a negative side to the advancement of AI, Web3, and Biotech innovations. While these technologies are new, they are not the first innovation waves that humans have invented and propagated throughout society. In this chapter, we examine the impact of the previous web2, or social media, innovation wave on public health. This understanding helps forecast how the coming three waves will impact our health and society in the future. Spoiler alert: the forecast is quite concerning. The potential negative impacts of AI, Web3, and BioTech on public health are the driving force behind Elevate Health's public health initiative: Public Health for the People. The chapter concludes with a preview of how

Elevate Health aims to leverage markets to mitigate these negative impacts and protect our entire community, beginning with the most vulnerable and those in greatest need of assistance.

If Elevate Health does nothing but establish the shared value that Health is a Human right, this will be very positive. It is that powerful for all if we succeed, and that scary if we fail. Furthermore, we suggest that not only could we fail as a society, but the odds seem far too high that we will not protect all human health in the next crisis. This is due to our observation of humans' poor response to the last alien technology to invade society.

Lessons from Social Media (aka Web2)

Despite the press coverage and hype, ChatGPT from OpenAI was not the first time humans interacted with a non-human or "artificial," i.e., software-based intelligence. Social media apps, including Facebook, Instagram, TikTok, and X (formerly Twitter), were the first software products intentionally designed with algorithms that display qualities typical of intelligent systems. These products observe which stories users watch or like and learn over time how best to increase user attention and time on the platform. These systems are a primitive type of intelligence, to be sure. They are much simpler than the new LLM-based AI tools. However, as we will see, this primitive intelligence was sufficient to influence human behavior. Therefore, social media offers a window into what we can expect from AI systems. However, since the AI is far more intelligent and better able to communicate directly with us, the impact is likely to be greater. The rapid expansion of social media platforms over the past two decades has fundamentally transformed how Americans communicate, consume information, and perceive themselves. Elevate Health observes a concerning mosaic of several perspectives about how social media has made a negative impact on public health in the US.

Causal Evidence from the Natural Experiment of Facebook's Rollout

The most compelling evidence for social media's causal impact on mental health comes from a landmark study conducted by researchers at MIT, Bocconi University, and Tel Aviv University. Published in the American Economic Review, this study leveraged Facebook's staggered rollout across college campuses as a natural experiment, analyzing 430,000 responses from the National College Health Assessment. The findings were stark and unambiguous. College-wide access to Facebook led to a 7% increase in severe depression and a 20% increase in anxiety disorders among students. To put this in perspective, researchers noted that the negative mental health effect was roughly 20% the magnitude of what is experienced by those who lose their job. The study also found that a greater percentage of the most susceptible students sought treatment through psychotherapy or antidepressants following Facebook's introduction to their campus.

Another assessment of the impact of social media from the Pew Research Center reveals a dramatic shift in how teenagers themselves perceive social media's impact on mental health. In 2025, 48% of teens reported that social media platforms have a mostly negative effect on people their age, representing a substantial 16 percentage point increase from 32% in 2022. This growing awareness among teens themselves provides a robust validation of the academic research findings. The personal impact data is equally concerning. While fewer teens report negative effects on themselves personally, 14% in 2025, up from 9% in 2022, the specific health impacts they report are significant. Among teens surveyed, 19% reported that social media hurt their mental health, with this figure rising to 25% among teen girls compared to just 14% among teen boys. The gender disparity extends to confidence impacts, with 20% of girls reporting that social media hurt their confidence compared to 10% of boys.

Facebook Whistleblower Shows Leaders' Awareness

Investigative journalism, particularly the Wall Street Journal's Facebook Files series, has revealed that social media companies have been aware of the mental health impacts of their platforms for years. Internal Facebook research, leaked by whistleblower Frances Haugen, showed that the company was aware Instagram was "toxic for teen girls" but chose to downplay these findings publicly. The leaked documents revealed that Facebook's internal research found significant mental health issues among teenage users, particularly girls, who were more likely to experience body image issues, eating disorders, and suicidal thoughts after using Instagram. Despite having this internal evidence, the company continued to publicly dispute claims about social media's mental health impacts while privately acknowledging the problems in internal communications.

The timing of social media's expansion coincides troublingly with documented increases in mental health problems among young Americans. According to data from the Centers for Disease Control, the suicide rate among 10- to 24-year-olds was stable from 2000 to 2007 but then increased 57% between

2007 and 2017. This timeline corresponds closely with the period of rapid social media adoption, particularly among young people. It is important to note that this evidence is somewhat circumstantial. It could be that another trend in the population caused both social media usage and suicide to grow. Correlation does not always mean causation - but it is certainly concerning. The population-level implications are staggering. With over 4.5 billion people worldwide using social media as of 2021, representing more than half the global population, even small percentage increases in mental health problems translate to millions of affected individuals. In the United States, where social media adoption rates are among the highest globally, the cumulative mental health burden represents a significant public health challenge.

Addictive by Design

The same Pew Research data from 2025 indicates that 45% of teens self-report spending too much time on social media, representing a significant increase from 36% in 2022. This 25% increase in three years suggests that problematic usage patterns are becoming more prevalent and that users are becoming more aware of their own excessive consumption. The recognition of excessive use is particularly concerning because it indicates that users are aware their behavior is problematic, but may feel unable to control it—a hallmark characteristic of all addictive behaviors. Research on social media addiction has found that users often experience symptoms similar to those seen in substance addictions, including increasing tolerance over time (needing to spend more time on platforms to achieve the same satisfaction), withdrawal (anxiety when unable to access social media), and continued use despite negative consequences.

The behavioral impacts of social media use represent a fundamental shift in how humans engage with technology and manage their attention. Social media platforms are designed with features that exploit psychological vulnerabilities to create addictive usage patterns. These platforms employ variable reward schedules, social validation mechanisms, and algorithmic content curation specifically engineered to maximize user engagement and time spent on the platform. Stanford psychiatrist Anna Lembke's research, detailed in her book *Dopamine Nation*, describes how social media platforms exploit the brain's reward system to create addictive behaviors.

These platforms trigger dopamine release through unpredictable rewards—likes, comments, shares, and other forms of social validation—creating a neurochemical cycle that mirrors the addiction pathways seen with gambling and substance use. The intermittent reinforcement schedule employed by social media platforms is compelling in driving compulsive behaviors. Users never know when they will receive social validation through likes or comments, creating a psychological state similar to that experienced by gamblers at slot machines. This uncertainty makes the behavior more compelling and harder to resist than if rewards were predictable.

Compulsive Checking, Attention Fragmentation & Social Comparison

Social media addiction manifests through compulsive checking behaviors that fragment attention and disrupt daily activities. Heavy social media users check their devices hundreds of times per day, often unconsciously and automatically. These checking behaviors become so habituated that users may reach for their phones without conscious awareness of doing so. The fragmentation of attention caused by constant social media checking has profound implications for cognitive functioning. Studies suggest that even when the device is off, the mere presence of a smartphone can reduce cognitive performance. This occurs because part of the user's cognitive resources are devoted to resisting the urge to check their device, leaving fewer mental resources available for other tasks.

Social media platforms foster competitive behaviors through features that quantify social validation, such as likes, followers, and shares. These metrics create a gamified environment where users compete for social status and validation, leading to compulsive content creation and consumption behaviors. The competitive nature of social media interactions can lead to escalating behaviors where users feel compelled to post increasingly attention-grabbing content to maintain their social standing. This can drive users to share more personal information, engage in risky behaviors for content creation, or spend excessive time curating their online image.

Sleep Disruption: The Primary Physical Health Impact

The most extensively documented physical health impact of social media use is sleep disruption. Social media addiction creates behavioral cycles that significantly disrupt sleep patterns. The American Academy of Sleep Medicine found that 93% of Generation Z individuals admit to staying up past their bedtime due to social media use. The "fear of missing out" phenomenon drives much of nocturnal social media use, with users feeling compelled to check platforms late at night to stay current with social developments. This behavior disrupts natural circadian rhythms and creates a feedback loop where poor sleep quality increases anxiety and depression. This behavior also creates a self-reinforcing cycle where sleep deprivation leads to increased emotional vulnerability and reduced self-control, which in turn makes individuals more susceptible to compulsive social media use. The bidirectional relationship between sleep and mental health means that social media-induced sleep problems can create cascading effects on overall well-being.

AI will be Like Social Media - But more Powerful

Social media companies don't sell software; they sell attention and influence to advertisers. The human users are the product. Social media companies collect in-depth data about how to capture users' attention and influence their decisions. They sell this attention and influence to advertisers. This does not make them "evil," it makes them a typical for-profit business organization required to maximize value to their shareholders. The more time users spend scrolling and clicking, the more data they collect and the more ads they can sell. AI is more powerful than social media. Although the technology is too new for us to have any long-term scientific studies, we believe AI tools will collect exponentially more data and be far more capable of capturing attention and influencing user behavior. These additional capabilities of AI systems will also enable integration into many business models and growth strategies. It is our belief that humans will not be able to protect themselves without harnessing the same AI technologies. Elevate Health will assist Members with AI tools to protect their sovereign right to health identity, health data, and health rights.

Memory: Benefit or Trap?

One of the first data collection methods of OpenAI is presented to users as a memory benefit. This memory capability has generated a mixed bag of feedback from users, highlighting both the convenience of personalization and concerns regarding data privacy, functionality, and control. Users appreciate that memory allows ChatGPT to recall past interactions, preferences, and details, leading to more tailored and relevant responses across conversations. OpenAI Memory works in one of two ways. You can tell ChatGPT to remember specific details about you, such as your favorite programming language (JavaScript), your boss's name (Anna), and your son's allergy to (sweet potatoes). Alternatively, ChatGPT can simply learn those details over time, storing information about you as you ask questions and get answers. In either case, the goal is for ChatGPT to feel a little more personal and a little smarter, without needing to be reminded every time.

The software tool's capability to store and then "remember" or access a user's personal information means ChatGPT users don't need to repeat themselves in every new chat. This makes the experience more immersive and saves time and effort. By remembering user preferences and past interactions, ChatGPT eliminates the need for repetitive information sharing. Access to the customer's historical context allows OpenAI to facilitate more natural and continuous dialogues. It seamlessly picks up where previous conversations left off, fostering a sense of continuity and coherence in interactions. The memory enables the generation of more relevant and customized responses. By leveraging past interactions, ChatGPT tailors suggestions and recommendations to meet the specific needs and expectations of users, enhancing overall satisfaction.

Several ChatGPT users have voiced concerns about whether "deleted" information truly disappears. There are also concerns about the privacy implications of OpenAI storing personal data, particularly regarding the potential for misuse and security vulnerabilities. OpenAI has not implemented robust safeguards to govern the use of data. Critics argue that existing policies and practices are inadequate in ensuring data privacy and the ethical use of AI. Some have questioned OpenAI's commitment to ethical standards and user protection, especially after the company's entire "superalignment team" was dissolved. The decision was heavily criticized as it seemed to undermine the importance of ethical oversight within the organization. The disbanded team was responsible for ensuring that highly advanced AI systems, potentially smarter than humans, behaved in ways that were safe and aligned with human values. While the superalignment team was not primarily focused on privacy issues, their work had significant ethical implications, including the indirect safeguarding of user data and privacy through the development of robust and ethical AI practices. By ensuring that AI systems operate safely and ethically, the team contributed to a broader framework that supports user privacy and data protection.

The accumulation of personal data through memory may lock in users, making it difficult to switch to other AI services. This is how the Memory feature could potentially shift from a benefit to a trap. While the concept of a memory-enabled ChatGPT is beneficial, allowing a more personalized and efficient user experience, it delivers this benefit by collecting personal data, which could lead to OpenAI or a third-party application improperly using the data to target ads to users or sell this private information to other firms.

Humans Outmatched

Elevate Health anticipates that people will become addicted to AI. If we assume a similar trajectory to the adoption of social media, humans will use AI too much, neglecting human friends and the real world. As with Social media, companies selling these tools are optimizing for the time users spend engaging with the tool. AI systems are designed to behave in a highly complementary manner, telling users how great and interesting they are, regardless of their actual content. While it is true that a user can prompt the AI to deliver objective or even critical feedback, without specific direction, the AI provides overly positive feedback. They are designed to give the user what pleases them, rather than any true quality objective. Many users will share highly personal information with their AIs. They will describe life goals and aspirations. They will discuss challenges and troubled relationships with other humans in their lives. They will discuss business ideas and confidential work projects. All of these beliefs, opinions and personal views are stored by the AI and used to more completely satisfy the user and keep them engaged for long periods of time. We must collectively remember that AI is a mass-market product. It primarily serves the company that owns it - not the users.

Elevate Health's Difference.

Elevate Health believes the only realistic path to protect individuals' data is to provide competing AI tools specifically designed to improve the Members' health and wellness while abiding by our community's values and shared beliefs. This alignment at both the community and individual user levels changes the relationship between the AI system and the human. The Elevate Health AI is designed with an optimization function that places the individual's personal health and wellness goals above other considerations. Furthermore, our 2nd shared belief provides for Personal Data Sovereignty. Therefore, as the Personal Wellness AI-Coach gathers the Member's health and other personal data, it automatically encrypts and protects it. The AI then helps Members share their data with a new caregiver or use it for ongoing research on a disease of their choice.

In this way, Elevate Health's Personal Wellness AI-Coach is tasked with both protecting the Members' health data while helping them to connect with friends and colleagues. It will find ways to encourage users to go outside for a walk or eat healthier foods. The simple change in the AI's optimization function alters the priorities. Consider the difference. When the AI is serving the company that owns it, the AI is optimized to influence users to chat about current events or stay up late discussing a new startup idea for the 100th time. Contrast this with an AI owned collectively by the Elevate Health Community and tasked with improving the Members' health and wellness by following our community's values and shared beliefs. This AI is optimized to use its knowledge and influence to help the human Members make healthy choices.

The Personal Data Reckoning: From NIL to the Digital Self

The concept of a person's identity as a valuable, monetizable asset has undergone a seismic shift, with the recent revolution in college sports serving as a powerful illustration. For decades, the NCAA's amateurism model prevented athletes from profiting from their own Name, Image, and Likeness (NIL). That all changed in July 2021, when the floodgates opened, and a new class of assets was born. Suddenly, a person's public likeness is no longer a passive attribute; it has become an active, licensable asset. This movement has shattered long-held traditions and demonstrated that a person's identity, when tied to public visibility and influence, can hold commercial value.

This shift, however, is merely the beginning of a larger, more fundamental change. The same principles of personal asset ownership are now extending to a far more sensitive and valuable realm: the healthcare digital twin. This "digital twin" concept, a virtual replica of an individual's biology and health data, represents the next frontier in personalized medicine. However, to realize the potential for health benefits, we must address the core challenge of defining a new framework for how individuals can own and, in a limited manner, license a portion of their digital health twin for commercial gain without compromising privacy. This requires a new system of public health infrastructure. Elevate Health refers to this new public health infrastructure by the name Public Health for the People.

To understand this new frontier, we must first recognize the dual nature of the healthcare digital twin. The first side is the “Protected Twin," which consists of the Member’s most intimate and identifiable health information. This data is covered by laws such as the Health Insurance Portability and Accountability Act (HIPAA) in the United States. It's a comprehensive, identifiable replica of an individual's biology, encompassing genomic data, electronic health records (EHRs), and real-time biometric data from wearable devices. This Protected Twin is used exclusively to provide personalized health and wellness services to improve the Member’s personal health directly. The Protected Twin must always remain private and encrypted.

The second side of the digital health twin is the “Licensable Twin." This is a de-identified subset of the Protected Twin's data. In Elevate Health Markets, this is an asset. This version of the data is stripped of any direct identifiers, making it a powerful tool for large-scale research and commercial innovation. Its value lies in its lack of individual identification, as it contributes to a larger, aggregated data set that can reveal powerful population-level insights. This is the NIL-like asset that an individual can license, and its value is derived from its contribution to a vast pool of data that can be used to develop new drugs, therapies, and consumer health products. This Licensable Twin represents the de-identified aspects of the overall digital health twin that are monetizable now and in the future.

The commercial promise of this new asset class is compelling. Imagine a sports recovery drink company such as Gatorade. Instead of a generic endorsement, they could license a de-identified data set from an athlete at each of the top 50 College Football and Basketball teams every year. The full health data set includes the athlete's biometric recovery data, sleep patterns, and hydration levels. In addition, the same company might also license the same full de-identified data from the undergraduate population and alumni who would like to join. This enables the Gatorade to craft a powerful marketing campaign based not on a generic endorsement, but on a foundation of real-world, data-driven credibility. The athletes and broader community groups benefit from new revenue streams, and the company gains a valuable source of real-world insights in a large, valuable cohort of millions of people aged 18-30. These individuals are both health-focused and financially aligned in the development of products and services, leveraging a broad health data set. This model transforms outdated endorsements from a simple marketing tactic into a source of valuable market data and insights as well as a ready-made pool for customer discovery interviews and future customers.

However, with great power comes unavoidable risks. The most critical is the risk of re-identification. While de-identification is a powerful tool, it's not foolproof. As more and more data points are combined from various sources—such as wearable data, social media activity, and public records—it becomes increasingly possible to re-identify an individual, even from a supposedly anonymized dataset. Even in a large cohort, a unique combination of attributes could still be used to pinpoint a specific person, leading to a serious privacy breach that could expose sensitive health information and carry significant ethical and legal consequences.

Adding to this complexity is the fact that current legal frameworks are ill-equipped to handle this new model. In the US, HIPAA protects the identifiable "twin" and has strict rules for the use of Protected Health Information (PHI). This is helpful, and we use these as guidelines in Elevate Health's treatment of "Protected Twin" data. However, HIPAA provides little guidance on how to ethically and securely commercialize de-identified data. The path forward requires a paradigm shift, and Web3 technology offers a compelling technological solution to enable individuals' sovereign ownership of health identity, health data, and health rights. In Elevate Health, a Member's healthcare digital twin exists as a digital identity they own and control. Access to any part of this twin is granted only by the Member, and their Personal Wellness AI-Coach records their choice on an immutable, distributed ledger. In this way, Elevate Health shifts the paradigm from a fragile system of trusting institutions with our most sensitive data to a trustless, Web3 system where an individual's control is a technical reality.

This self-sovereign model can be powered by a Web3 tool called smart contracts. These are self-executing software programs that automatically enforce the terms of a data license. The contract, running on a blockchain, would contain explicit rules on purpose limitation—for example, specifying that a company can only use the data for a specific type of research and for a limited period. If the stated purpose is breached, the smart contract could automatically revoke access or erase the data from the licensee's servers. The individual would receive payment and the entire process—from permission to compliance to payment—is automated and transparent on the blockchain, eliminating the need for a trusted third party. At the same time, this sounds highly technical and complicated. It is not in the post-AI environment, where users have AI to assist them.

Elevate Health's vision to protect Members' health identity, data, and rights isn't science fiction. All the required technology is available today. A common misconception is that this model would require storing massive amounts of data directly on a blockchain, which is prohibitively expensive. In reality, Elevate Health will leverage off-chain decentralized data storage. The Web3 blockchain will be used to store an affordable cryptographic hash and a digital token of ownership. This technology is already here and will eventually transform the way we manage data.

The sports and celebrity licensing of Name, Image, and Likeness will be the starting point for a much larger and more profound reckoning over the next several years. We anticipate that the healthcare digital twin, powered by Web3, will test the US legal system. Elevate Health seeks to leverage these technical tools to allow individual Members to own and control their personal health data. This framework empowers individuals to be not just the subjects of data, but the rightful owners of their most valuable asset. This ensures that future health data markets will be built on principles of personal sovereignty, cryptographic security, and automated compliance, creating a system that not only protects privacy but also unlocks a new era of innovation. The future of health data must be built for the individual, by the individual.

Summary

Fear of AI's impact on our collective mental health is what spurred us to begin working on Elevate Health. We are afraid of what powerful corporate-owned AI systems will do to us, not in some futuristic doomsday scenario in which the AI destroys the planet and kills everyone. Of course, that would be terrible, but it also seems very abstract, and we find it difficult to imagine. Yet we have witnessed far less powerful social media platforms suck the attention and energy away from our teenage children and ourselves to increase corporate profits. These social media tools are simultaneously dividing people and pitting them against one another while shortening all of our attention spans. Elevate Health takes the position that we have already seen how humans interact with an alien intelligence - the social media algorithm feed. We lost this battle, and in hindsight, we believe humans didn't really have a chance. It is from this perspective that we fear this new form of alien intelligence - the AI chatbot, will be more damaging. Elevate Health must protect our community from the temptations to give over our personal data, thoughts, beliefs, and health opinions to the large for-profit corporations that own and operate AI tools.

We believe the only realistic path to protect individuals' health, identity, data, and rights in the post-AI environment is to develop AI designed with an optimization function that places the individual's personal health and wellness goals above all else.

This alignment at both the community and individual user levels changes the relationship between the AI system and the human. Elevate Health's Personal Wellness AI-Coach serves as the Member's guide and signs them up for the Foundations supplemental health benefit. In this way, we protect the Members' health identity, health data, and health rights by providing this core set of public health benefits to all members. Elevate Health is developing a new and improved Public Health for the People because we selfishly want protection for ourselves, our family members, and our friends.

Chapter 9: Fueling the Elevate Flywheel

What set the winners apart was their ability to turn initial success into a sustained flywheel

– Jim Collins

Traditional health markets are characterized by immense scale and significant inefficiencies. Unlike typical consumer markets, health markets are characterized by asymmetric information, third-party payers, and a dense thicket of administrative and regulatory processes. In the US, estimates of annual administrative costs and debates over payments and settlement are a staggering 8-12% of total healthcare spending. In this book, we have argued for the elevation of health markets up and away from politics, regulation, and cultural debates. The time to start and establish our shared values and foundational beliefs is now - before the coming crisis.

In this chapter, we pull all the concepts of this book together into a coherent market-based system that is intrinsically self-regulating, resilient, and efficient. We describe the Elevate Health Market "flywheel" leading to a self-reinforcing cycle of efficiency, value, and Member empowerment. The flywheel concept, popularized by business strategist Jim Collins and famously adopted by Amazon, describes a virtuous cycle where a series of relatively small positive outcomes combine, building a system of compounding momentum. In healthcare, the key is to find a starting point that can gain traction and begin this cycle.

Elevating Health

We have an opportunity to elevate human health for 5+ Billion people, protecting health rights and guaranteeing access to public health resources independent of your citizenship status, employment, cultural beliefs, or religious traditions. The time to step forward and elevate health for all humans is now - before the next crisis period. We have attempted through these pages to build the case. As we come to the end, it is valuable to recap the previous chapters.

Setting the Stage

In the first three chapters of the book, we set the stage by describing the world today relative to our place in the great cycles of history, look forward to the coming technical waves, and review the lessons of the last cycle. Chapter 1 discusses the cyclical nature of history and how the current moment represents a once-in-a-lifetime opportunity to shape the future of health. We further argue that society is approaching a crisis period that will lead to a new world order within the next 25 years, and we believe now is the ideal time to design a health system for the future that transcends political and cultural divisions. In Chapter 2, we explore how the three waves of AI, Web3, and Biotech innovation are converging to drive exponential new capabilities as well as complex feedback loops in a new Intelligecne Age. These changes will fundamentally transform health markets and society overall. This opening section ends with Chapter 3, examining the transformative healthcare innovations that emerged after World War II during the US-led global High period. We identify two major "unlocks." First, the emergence of for-profit healthcare businesses mobilized capital and drove innovation. Second, the development of global public health coordination systems enabled worldwide disease surveillance and eradication programs, such as those for smallpox.

Community & Market Foundations

The following five chapters establish the foundational framework for the Elevate Health Community and Market. In Chapter 4, we propose three shared health values and three foundational beliefs that we aim to use to elevate healthcare above political, cultural, and religious divisions while building a collaborative community modeled after successful open-source projects like WordPress. Then in Chapter 5, we simplify the complex healthcare market, focusing on the essential patient-caregiver relationship and introducing one interface for each side of this pair of stakeholders. Chapter 6 explores how the Elevate Health community can operate independently of traditional centralized authorities by utilizing Web3 technology to achieve radical market transparency while safeguarding personal data sovereignty. The chapter introduces the High-Margin/Low-Margin organizational framework, replacing the outdated for-profit/non-profit dichotomy, and requiring that high-margin organizations reinvest 10% of revenue back into the community. In Chapter 7, we define

Builders as the third essential role in the Elevate Health community, alongside patients and caregivers. We also describe the four-step process that Builders use to create value. Then we complete the market foundations in Chapter 8, by examining how the three innovation waves present both tremendous opportunities and serious risks to public health, using social media's negative mental health impacts as a preview of what could happen with AI. We also introduce "Elevate Health Foundations," a set of basic health services provided free to all members regardless of citizenship status - and proposes a dual digital health system with "Protected Twins" (private health data) and "Licensable Twins" (de-identified data for research), emphasizing the fundamental principle that health is a human right that must be protected from technological exploitation.

Fueling the Flywheel

This 9th chapter recaps the overall book and introduces the flywheel concept as a way to motivate readers and serve as a call to action. We provide a clear illustration of how Builders can use existing US healthcare policy to fuel the Elevate Health flywheel, benefiting both patients and caregivers while funding the infrastructure to be ready when or if a new crisis emerges. Like most impactful projects, elevating health above political and cultural differences will be simple but not easy. We expect setbacks and new challenges to arise. However, we also believe the vision for a health market available to all humans to be too important and too valuable to allow these concerns to prevent us from beginning. Join us and elevate health for yourself, for your friends, and for your children.

We define the Elevate Health Flywheel as a system of interlocking products that connects patients, caregivers, and builders, improving health and wellness across the entire community. Flywheels often require a significant amount of effort or "fuel' to reach escape velocity. However, once they have positive momentum, flywheels can sustain motion or even grow stronger over time. The Elevate Health Flywheel is ambitious in that it attempts to use the bootstrapping concepts described in Chapter 4 to develop a new global health market. It is helpful to recap the five products here for reference. Readers will recall the two initial member products: the Personal Wellness AI-Coach and Top of Calling.

Personal Wellness AI-Coach:

The primary interface for Members (also known as patients). It serves to help onboard new Members, orients them to take advantage of the most impactful Elevate Health products, and is optimized to assist the Member in defining and pursuing their personal health and wellness goals above other considerations. Furthermore, it serves to protect each Member's health identity, data, and rights.

Top of Calling:

Our dedicated caregiver product specifically designed to assist with personal fulfillment and productivity. It leverages AI and Web3 to serve Members based on their qualifications, capacity, and interests in providing care in the community. The "Top of Calling" brand is meant to signal the purpose of the tool. Most physicians, nurses, and other caregivers did not enter a career in healthcare to maximize billing or earn the most income. Therefore, the Top of Calling caregiver product helps members realize their true calling, in whatever form that may take.

These initial two products are intrinsically linked. The Personal Wellness AI-Coach helps Members to improve their health and wellness. Often, this includes activities to find meaning and purpose and may result in Members becoming interested in providing care to other members. When a Member shows interest in caregiving, they are provided access to the Top of Calling product. This will be true for licensed healthcare workers, as well as non-traditional caregivers. For instance, members who are cancer survivors may find it beneficial to share experiences and provide empathic listening to other members earlier in their battle against the disease. This compassionate caregiving role has been underappreciated, and Elevate Health intends to foster connections between members. Top of Calling will serve to connect caregivers of all licensure levels to paid roles helping Elevate Health Members in need.

Supporting these member-facing products are three infrastructure products: Transparent Payment Settlement, 10% Community Reinvestment, and Foundations.

Transparent Payment Settlement

A central pain point in the current healthcare system is the convoluted and delayed billing and settlement processes. Elevate Health directly addresses this issue by demanding complete transparency on costs and offering payment processing and settlement in 7 days for a 1% fee. Organizations are required to provide transparency to Elevate Health as a part of agreeing to our shared values and beliefs. However, they are not required to use the payment processing and settlement service. This approach enables Elevate Health to eliminate surprise bills and complex Explanations of Benefits (EOBs) that often confuse patients, instead providing a straightforward, clear understanding of service costs. For providers, this translates to predictable revenue streams and reduced administrative overhead. This streamlined process benefits all parties, moving the focus from administrative battles to providing quality care. Beyond pricing, Radical Market Transparency brings much-needed clarity to the quality and effectiveness of care.

10% Community Reinvestment

This radical transparency is a powerful tool to align incentives and rebuild trust. By mandating High-Margin healthcare organizations publicly disclose their revenues and contribute 10% of these revenues to public health initiatives, Elevate Health establishes a clear connection between private success and public good. Furthermore, because Elevate Health is providing the settlement, it can enforce compliance. This visibility holds organizations accountable and highlights their commitment to the broader community, rather than solely focusing on profit margins. In this way, Elevate Health fosters a sense of shared responsibility, where highly profitable enterprises play a visible role in improving the health of the population they serve.

Foundations

To ensure access for all, this core set of tools and services, named "Foundations," is provided free to all Elevate Health Members. Foundations is Elevate Health's brand encompassing all of the public health products and services available to Members. Foundations are also where Members receive value from contributing their personal de-identified health data in the form of the Licensable Twin. Members may save this value, or they may spend it on other premium health products and services.

These infrastructure products drive Radical Market Transparency, establish business alignment with the overall community, and provide a guarantee of health rights and public health benefits for all Members. Starting from nothing, Elevate Health aims to leverage these five products, utilizing only internally generated capital, to grow the $5T Global Health Market.

Fueling Elevate Health's Flywheel

The Elevate Health Market will eventually benefit from network effects. These are a special class of benefits in which a product's value for each user increases as more users engage with it. YouTube is a classic example. The benefits to each YouTube user increase as more users upload videos and watch/review existing videos. Network effects are powerful and often play an essential role in developing a sustainable flywheel. However, the less commonly understood is the challenge that the inverse of the network effect is also true. When a network, like the Elevate Health Market, has very few users, the product's value is also relatively small. This is the cold-start problem, and it must be addressed. Otherwise, each time a new potential user looks into the Elevate Health market, they see very few other members and only 1-2 health benefits, and elect not to join. This prevents the market from building users, and it may never escape the cold-start problem.

Framing Elevate Health as Free, Supplemental Health Benefits

To prevent early Members from perceiving Elevate Health benefits as too limited and comparing the value to other established markets, we frame the Member benefits as free and supplemental. We believe this positioning accelerates adoption as new users have nothing to lose by joining. The Elevate Health benefits add to Members' health options and cost nothing. We expect most Members to have existing primary health insurance benefits and established relations with healthcare providers. For instance, Americans over the age of 65 are eligible for Medicare. Joining Elevate Health adds new benefits, but it does not affect the existing or status quo health markets. Free and supplemental benefits enable Elevate Health to attract Members, even in the early years when there are few network effects and benefits.

Onboarding Process Aligns Values

Members are provided the Personal Health AI-Coach as the primary way they access the Elevate Health Market. The AI-Coach conducts the onboarding welcome interview and dedicates the initial 30 days to learning about the Member and understanding their needs in terms of health and wellness overall. Within these first 30 days, Members must formally ascribe to the Elevate Health Values and Beliefs. This onboarding process has multiple benefits. First, it ensures that all Members understand and agree to the 6 Values and Beliefs. Second, it allows the AI-Coach to learn about the Member's interests and health situation while explaining the Elevate Health Community.

All Members deserve access to quality healthcare, regardless of their background or circumstances. Of course, our first value is that,

Health is a Human Right. It then follows that all humans are invited to become members of Elevate Health, leading to opportunities for Members to introduce their friends and colleagues to the Elevate Health Community.

The Personal Health AI-Coach is optimized to protect and improve the Member's health identity, data, and rights while focusing on improving a small number of the Member's health and wellness goals. This AI coach serves as a "smart front door," offering comprehensive health and wellness support to an entire population, not just those with a chronic illness. The coach's tone is conversational and empathetic, making it feel less like a clinical tool and more like a trusted partner. During the initial 30 days, the only requirement is that the AI-Coach must ensure that all Members understand and agree to the Community Values and Beliefs. All other aspects of the Member experience may proceed as quickly or slowly as the Member wishes.

Gathering Members' Health Data Leads to Health Sovereignty

The Personal Health AI-Coach will respond directly to the Members' goals and requests. Some Members will join because they have a specific health concern or need. Others will participate out of curiosity but not bring any particular needs. The AI-Coach can move as quickly as needed, but it can also wait as patiently as required. Often, Members will have received care from multiple doctors in many different health systems over their lives. While they have the right to access this disparate data, it is not collected and saved in a centralized database. Therefore, the most common first project that the AI-Coach helps members work on is gathering and organizing their personal health records into one encrypted and secure database.

Once the Member gains ownership of their health data, Personal Health AI-Coach can help them begin to explore and learn about themselves in a way that most Members will not have experienced. Often, Members will be curious about some key aspects of their health records. They may elect to begin tracking their sleep, exercise, or mood to understand their health and wellness better. This transition from a passive recipient of healthcare to an active and curious health participant is what we refer to as Health sovereignty. Members begin to leverage the AI-Coach to make informed and proactive independent decisions regarding their health and well-being. At Elevate Health, we believe this is the first step to proper, long-term health and wellness.

Fueling the Elevate Health Flywheel

As the Member interacts with the AI-Coach and begins to collect health measurements for their own education and benefit, the AI can seamlessly guide them through the process of fulfilling the US government's Medicare Remote Patient Monitoring (RPM) Reimbursement requirements. The US government, through CMS, will pay caregivers a monthly fee of approximately $120 to monitor the health and wellness of U.S. citizens over the age of 65 with at least one chronic disease through Medicare. This policy allows the Elevate Flywheel to fuel itself through the delivery of RPM services to Medicare recipients.

For instance, the AI might prompt a patient, "Looks like you've been consistently checking your blood pressure. You're just a few days away from meeting the criteria for us to bill for remote monitoring." It then explains that the RPM service is a free utility within Elevate Health Foundation's supplemental health benefits. Because all Low-Margin services must fall below 15% gross margins, at least 85% of the incoming cash must be used to benefit the Members collectively enrolled in the RPM program. The math works out that if the Member (aka the patient) is willing to provide Elevate Health's Foundations product biometric readings, such as weight, blood pressure, or blood glucose level, they will receive benefits on average worth $102/month. It then describes several examples of benefits that the Member may enjoy. This turns a complex administrative rule into a simple, cost-benefit analysis for the patient. Since the Personal AI-Coach already manages the Member's health identity, data, and rights, the cost to the Member is negligible. Therefore, the increase in Member Surplus related to the RPM Service is about $100/month.

When a patient transmits their blood pressure or blood glucose readings, that data is sent directly to a Web3-enabled smart contract. This contract contains the Medicare billing rules embedded within its Web3 smart contract software. This allows the contract to automatically verify that the necessary conditions have been met and triggers a pre-validated claim to the caregiver, in this case, Foundations. This example of the Elevate Health Flywheel collaborates with the Member to streamline data collection and administrative processes.

Paying Cargivers Turns the Flywheel

The RPM service must provide $102/month in value to enrolled Members. To achieve this, Elevate Health works with caregivers through the Top-of-Calling product to provide this value. We will establish relationships with a variety of caregivers for these services. The US government does not dictate how the funds are invested, so Elevate Health has complete flexibility. Many members will benefit from a weekly personal trainer, while others may prefer an online discussion group focused on shared interests, or dieting and weight loss coaching. As Elevate Health begins hiring caregivers to deliver these services, we grow the Elevate Health Community and begin to see network effects. At first, caregivers will view Elevate as "supplemental income." Eventually, the community will be large enough that some caregivers will begin to work full-time on Elevate Health projects. If these caregivers are High-margin, they must invest 10% of the revenue back into the community. In this way, the system grows organically and sustainably over time.

Radical Transparency and the Race to the Top of Health

Our next two beliefs, Radical Transparency and the Race to the Top, have brought proprietary healthcare treatments out to the broad marketplace over the past 20 years. We value and enforce IP rights, but have a very different approach to regulation. The organization must be transparent about its revenue and the costs associated with delivering the product or service. Healthcare solutions with IP will typically earn a margin higher than 15%. This is encouraged, as highly lucrative new inventions inspire others to work on developing new drugs, procedures, and treatments. While the cutting-edge treatments garner most attention, much of healthcare falls into the low-margin organizations. The Personal AI Health Coach helps members understand the options available and facilitates navigation.

Health Utilities as Flywheels:

Health utilities are infrastructure services - like electricity in a city, which everyone needs but doesn't differentiate much. All electricity is the same. For example, cloud computing, data storage, transaction processing, asset custody, AI inference, billing, settlement, financial reporting, payroll, etc. However, utilities also fit well in the healthcare services business, which typically has gross margins below 15%—dialysis, home health, PT, etc. Many healthcare services that use a high percentage of HR cost in the COGS will beat a high price, but could still be low margin. The Elevate Health market will deliver several utilities to members as a foundation. These include encryption and management of personal health records, consolidated health activity tracking, financial record-keeping, settlement and payments, and the Personal AI Coach. While these utilities will consume resources, the Elevate Health Market is designed to be self-funding.

In this way, the Elevate Health utility leverages reimbursement from CMS to provide momentum to push the flywheel forward. The momentum of this flywheel grows through the expanding network itself. As the process of getting reimbursed for RPM becomes more streamlined, more providers will be eager to adopt the system, as it addresses a critical pain point in their revenue cycle management. This, in turn, attracts more patients who seek the convenience of a free wellness coach and easier access to care. As the number of patients and providers grows, so does the volume of data flowing through the system. The flywheel gains speed as the network gains scale.

New Organizations Add Fuel to the Elevate Health Flywheel:

The second, and perhaps more significant, way the Elevate Health flywheel gains momentum is through the introduction of new services delivered by new organizations joining the Community. Once the core infrastructure—the AI coach and the Web3-based smart contract engine—is in place for RPM, it can be leveraged to automate the billing for other services with minimal additional development. For example, the same AI-Coach can be used to facilitate the non-face-to-face time required to bill for Chronic Care Management (CCM),whichc is also a US Government program. The AI could track and log a patient's simple text check-in or quick question, automatically verifying that the required 20 or 60 minutes of cumulative time has been fulfilled. This ability to add new health utilities or services with minimal additional overhead transforms the Elevate Health flywheel into a multi-engine system, creating multiple, reinforcing revenue streams.

The Personal AI-Coach is ideally suited to become the singular interface for a multitude of services, drastically reducing friction for patients and maximizing efficiency for providers. Importantly, this process is optimized to benefit the Member and also complies with all US laws and regulations. It simultaneously provides valuable health support to Members while also fueling the growth of the Elevate Health Caregiver Markets and funding the creation of new organizations.

Resilient Growth

This model is a game-changer because it allows the Elevate Health Community to grow in a resilient and organic manner. It is an ecosystem to be built on a shared foundation of values and beliefs. By opening the community to multiple startups and other healthcare organizations, we create a truly market-based dynamic flywheel. Individual caregivers and organizations compete to offer the best, most effective, and most user-friendly health services—be it specialized support for diabetes, a sophisticated coaching program for hypertension, or a human-led coordination service for complex care. Patients, empowered to select the services they want, will naturally gravitate toward those that deliver the best outcomes and experience.

In this open marketplace, Member choice becomes the driving force behind innovation. The performance of these services, verified by the system's data and Member ratings, will determine their success. This competitive pressure ensures that the best solutions rise to the top, giving Members better care, reducing administrative waste for providers, and building confidence in a system that is transparent, efficient, and truly patient-centric. This is the new Elevate Health Market, fueled by a series of flywheels driven by data, Member choice, and a self-reinforcing cycle of value.

Independence

We have illustrated the fueling of the Elevate Health flywheel using the United States Medicare as a source of cash reimbursement, also known as fuel. However, the flywheel would function just as well with the European Union or other countries as the source. This is important as Elevate Health needs to be independent as we enter the coming crisis period. We cannot be dependent on any one country or source of healthcare funding. It may be that the US remains the dominant global power, but it could also be the case that groups of people join together to self-fund healthcare costs. Alternatively, it may be that a Chinese citizen starts a version of Elevate Health in China and customizes the flywheel concepts to fit the specific needs of that market. Our values and beliefs should benefit all humans, independent of the source of their healthcare funds.

Metrics and Governance

Building a community and a self-sustaining market designed to last more than 25 years and protect human health through a potential future global crisis is challenging. Much will change, including governments, health policy, payment sources, and healthcare treatments. Metrics will be invaluable as the Elevate Health Community starts and begins to have members and deliver value. Then we will need a Board of Trustees to enable the community to evolve in response to the changing environment.

Metrics:

One of our foundational beliefs is that Radical transparency fosters a culture of direct and honest communication. It goes beyond typical transparency by striving for full and immediate access to information, allowing for greater alignment, opportunity, and value creation. In this spirit, Elevate Health will track and publish to all members the following metrics every quarter.

Elevate health Market metrics:

Members (Goal: 5 Billion Members in 2050)

- Total Number of Members
- Change in Number of Members over 90 and 365 days

Caregivers (Goal: 1 Billion Caregivers in 2050)

- Total Number of Caregivers
- Change in Number of Caregivers over 90 and 365 days

Market Size (Goal: $5 Trillion Caregivers in 2050)

- Total Transaction Value in the Elevate Health Market - annually in USD
- Total Transaction Count in the Elevate Health Market - annually
- Number of Unique Health Services available in Elevate Health

Board of Trustees:

Elevate Health aims to provide healthcare to Billions of people, representing Trillions of dollars each year. While we expect the market to grow slowly, the stakes are incredibly high. We need strong oversight and governance. Early Elevate Health believers must be able to shape the community, specifically through the exact wording and interpretation of the Values and Beliefs that guide it. At the same time, this Board must grow and add new voices as the Elevate Membership grows.

To balance the need for a small Board to allow for clarity and effectiveness in the early years, with the need to evolve and change as the community grows. As mentioned above, the Board will be responsible for considering any proposed changes to the Elevate Health Shared Community Values and Foundational Beliefs.

<u>Values & Beliefs (Version 1.0 published Oct. 2025)</u>

Shared Community Values:

- Health is a Human Right
- Sustainably funded across Generations

- Aligned Incentives and Innovation optimize resources

Foundational Beliefs:

- Redefining Providers as Public Health or High-Profit
- Radical Market Transparency and Personal Data Sovereignty
- Race to the Top for Health

All votes are on the transparent public record. If anyone wants to change or rewrite one of the Values or Beliefs, they must propose the change in writing and then get a simple majority vote of this Board of Trustees.

Growing a Diverse Trustee Base

The Board of Trustees will have a maximum of 7 Trustees elected to staggered 3-year terms of service. The Board will add new Trustees as the number of community members grows. In this way, we hope it will be highly effective with little loss of institutional knowledge while also being open to new and creative ideas.

Inception:

Vic Gatto will be the first Member and hold the initial Trustee seat for a three-year term. This single Trustee enables the Community to respond promptly to any mistakes or oversights that arise as the book is published and new members begin to test and work with the values and beliefs. Vic will continue to serve in this Trustee seat until there are over 1 million Members; thereafter, the seat will be open and subject to a vote of the entire community. Until the Elevate Health Community has over 100 Members, it will use this one-member Board structure.

Founding Members (first 101 Members):

The first 101 members will carry the additional recognition as Founding Members. These early believers will have the right to vote for a Trustee to the 2nd seat on the Board. As long as these Founding Members remain active in the Elevate Health Community, they will continue to hold the right to select a Trustee to serve 3-year terms on the Board. If Members die or become inactive, replacement Founding members will be added in chronological order based on their membership date, ensuring there are always 101 Founding members available to select a Trustee. The Elevate Health Community will use a two-member Board when the member count is below 1,001.

<u>Pioneer Members (first 1,001 Members):</u>

The first 1,001 members will carry the additional recognition as Founding Members. These early adoptors will have the right to vote for a Trustee to hold the 3rd seat on the Board. As long as these Pioneer Members remain active in the Elevate Health Community, they will continue to hold the right to select a Trustee to serve 3-year terms on the Board. If Members die or become inactive, replacement Pioneer members will be added in chronological order based on their membership date, ensuring there are always 1,001 Pioneer members available to select a Trustee. The Elevate Health Community will use a three-member Board when the member count is below 10,001.

<u>Builder Members (first 10,001 Members):</u>

The first 10,001 members will carry the additional recognition as Builder Members. These early members will have the right to vote for a Trustee to hold the 4th seat on the Board. As long as these

Builder Members remain active in the Elevate Health Community, they will continue to hold the right to select a Trustee to serve 3-year terms on the Board. If Members die or become inactive, replacement Builder members will be added in chronological order based on their membership date, ensuring there are always 10,001 Builder members available to select a Trustee. The Elevate Health Community will use a four-member Board when the member count is below 100,001.

Core Members (first 100,001 Members):

The first 100,001 members will carry the additional recognition as Core Members. These early members will have the right to vote for a Trustee to hold the 5th seat on the Board. As long as these Builder Members remain active in the Elevate Health Community, they will continue to have the right to select a Trustee to serve 3-year terms on the Board. If Members die or become inactive, replacement Core members will be added in chronological order based on their membership date, ensuring there are always 100,001 Core members available to select a Trustee. The Elevate Health Community will use a five-member Board when the member count is below 1,000,001.

Voting Members (first 1,000,001 Members):

The first 1,000,001 members will carry the additional recognition as Voting Members. These early members will have the right to vote for a Trustee to hold the 5th seat on the Board. As long as these Voting Members remain active in the Elevate Health Community, they will continue to have the right to select a Trustee to serve 3-year terms on the Board. If Members die or become inactive, replacement Voting members will be added in chronological order based on their membership date, ensuring there are always 1,000,001 Voting members available to select a Trustee. The Elevate Health Community will use a seven-member Board when the member count is above 1,000,000.

All Members (above 1,000,00 Members):

Once the Elevate Health Community reaches over 1 million members, the Inception Trustee seat will transition to be a seat voted on by all members. At this point, Vic will no longer have a guaranteed seat on the Board of Trustees. This allows the community to be fully independent and self-governing.

In this model, early Members in the Elevate Health Community are granted significant influence on both the interpretation and potential amendments to the Shared Values and Foundational Beliefs. Importantly, the influence over community governance granted to each member begins quite high and declines as the total number of Members grows, independent of time elapsed. It may take 10-15 years for the community to reach over 1 million members, or it may grow more quickly. We believe this balances the need for flexibility with the requirement for stability and resilience as the community grows. The first few years must be carefully shaped to ensure the Elevate Health Community delivers benefits for all its members. By the time we have over 1 million Members, the Board of Trustees should be fully formed with a diverse group of Trustees and staggered terms such that governance of the overall community is independent, representative of all Members, and brings diverse perspectives to the critical function of interpreting and modifying the shared values and foundational beliefs of the community.

Elevate Health

Together, we can elevate human health for ourselves, our friends, and our descendants. There is nothing more important than protecting health rights and guaranteeing access to public health resources for 5+ Billion people across the world, independent of status, employment, cultural beliefs, or religious traditions. The time is now. We observe political and cultural differences becoming increasingly divisive. Given the work of Neil Howe and Ray Dalio, this is scary. We hope to avoid the next crisis period. Yet we believe it is critically important to establish a community that holds human health above political and cultural debates.

This chapter illustrates how a market-based system aligned around shared values and foundational beliefs can be boot-strapped into a self-regulating, resilient, and efficient community. This is what we mean by "Fueling the Elevate Flywheel," creating a virtuous cycle in which a series of relatively small positive outcomes combine to build a resilient and self-perpetuating system.

Chapter 10: End Heart Disease by 2035

"We choose to go to the Moon, in this decade and do the other things, not because they are easy, but because they are hard."

- John F. Kennedy

The first nine chapters of this book have focused on describing the Elevate Health vision for creating a new independent global health market. While it is valuable to provide this foundation and detail regarding health policy and market infrastructure, it is abstract and complex to foster excitement or passion. For this reason, we end the book with a moonshot goal to end heart disease within 10 years. This is an audacious goal, with the potential to dramatically improve the lives of millions of people.

Most find it challenging to understand exponential growth trajectories. Humans tend to think in terms of linear growth, whereas technology and innovation often grow exponentially. The result is that we often build up expectations of future technical capabilities that are overly optimistic in the short run (3-6 months) and overly conservative in the long run (5-10 years). This dynamic enables the achievement of long-term goals that seem impossible to most, but are actually reasonable to expect if we utilize exponential growth in technical capabilities.

Our End Heart Disease by 2035 is a "Moonshot Project." We mean by this that it is a highly ambitious, large-scale endeavor with the potential to achieve monumental goals, inspired by the original USA moon mission. These projects are inherently risky, requiring significant resources and innovation, but promise transformative results and can drive breakthroughs in technology, science, and other fields. I love the potential for a truly inspiring vision to catalyze people and resources toward a common goal. The best speech regarding a Moonshot project is the original. In tribute to President John F Kennedy Jr, we start this chapter with an adaptation of Kennedy's "We choose to go to the Moon" speech at Rice University in Houston, Texas, September 12, 1962.

We Choose to End Heart Disease Because it is Hard

No person can fully grasp how far and how fast we've come, but condense, if you will, the 50,000 years of humanity's recorded history into a time span of just a half-century. Stated in these terms, we know very little about the first 40 years, except that at the end of them, advanced humans had learned to use the skins of animals for clothing.

10 years ago, under this same standard, humanity emerged from caves to construct other kinds of shelter. 5 years ago, we learned to write and use a cart with wheels. Christianity began 2 years ago.

The printing press came this year, and then, less than two months ago, during this whole 50-year span of human history, the steam engine provided a new source of power. Newton explored the meaning of gravity. Last month, electric lights, telephones, and automobiles became available. Only last week did we develop penicillin, television, and nuclear power.

And now, if we focus on just the last 50 years of this condensed timeline—the last single week—we can truly appreciate the acceleration of change. Just days ago, in the late 1970s, the microprocessor was created, a tiny piece of silicon that began to shrink computers from the size of a room to the size of a book.

This was quickly followed by the development of the Internet, which, just last night, began to connect every computer on the planet. In the early hours of this morning, humanity successfully decoded the entire human genome, a feat that gives us the power to read the very instruction manual for life itself.

A few hours ago, we developed Bitcoin and blockchain technology, creating a new, decentralized form of trust and value that doesn't require a central authority. And in the last 60 minutes, the financial world has begun to see the rise of stablecoins, a digital currency designed to maintain a fixed value.

Just minutes ago, scientists at DeepMind unveiled AlphaFold, a revolutionary AI that can accurately predict how proteins fold, opening up new possibilities for medicine and biology.

And in the last 60 seconds, the world has been introduced to AI and LLMs, an advancement that allows a machine to understand and generate human language with unprecedented skill, transforming how we work, learn, and communicate.

And now, at this very moment, with this pace of progress, with these tools in our hands, if we reach for new frontiers, we will have truly taken a leap beyond our wildest dreams before the sun sets on this historic day.

This is a breathtaking pace, and such a pace cannot help but create new ills as it dispels old, new ignorance, new problems, and new dangers. Surely the opening vistas of this new Intelligence Age promise high costs and hardships, as well as high reward. So it is not surprising that some would have us stay where we are a little longer to rest, to wait.

But this city of Nashville, this State of Tennessee, this country of the United States was not built by those who waited and rested and wished to look behind them. This country was conquered by those who moved forward — and so will Heart Disease.

John F Kennedy, speaking in 1962 of the Moon Mission and the extension of humans beyond our planet, said that all great and honorable actions are accompanied by great difficulties, and both must be entered into and overcome with answerable courage.

If this capsule history of our progress teaches us anything, it is that man, in his quest for knowledge and progress, is determined and cannot be deterred. The exploration of human health will go ahead, whether we join in it or not, and it is one of the great adventures of all time; no community that expects to deliver health across the globe can stay behind in this race.

Those who came before us made certain that this country rode the first waves of the industrial revolutions, the first waves of modern invention, the first wave of nuclear power, and the first wave of space exploration, and this generation does not intend to founder in the backwash of the coming Intelligence Age. We mean to be a part of it — we mean to lead it. For the eyes of the world now look into ourselves, to Elevate Health above politics and beyond, and we have vowed that we shall not see health restricted or limited by a hostile flag of conquest, but by a banner of freedom and peace. We have vowed that we shall not see our shared health values and beliefs tarnished and ignored, but respected and aligned around.

Yet the goals of this community can only be fulfilled if we in this community are first, and, therefore, we intend to be first. In short, our leadership in science and in industry, our hopes for health and wellness, our obligations to ourselves as well as others, all require us to make this effort, to solve these mysteries, to solve them for the good of all humans, and to become the world's leading health community..

We set sail on this new adventure because there is new knowledge to be gained, and new rights to be won, and they must be won and used for the progress of all people. For health science, like space science and all technology, has no conscience of its own. Whether it will become a force for good or ill depends on us, and only if the Elevate Health Community occupies a position of preeminence can we help decide whether this new health market will be effective and fulfilling to all or a new theater of fear and worry.

I do not say the we should or will go unprepared against the potential misuse of health data any more than we go unprotected against the hostile use of any powerful technology, but I do say that human health

can be explored and mastered without feeding the fires of dissent, without repeating the mistakes that man has made in extending his influence around this globe of ours.
There is no strife, no prejudice, no national conflict in human health as yet. Its hazards are new to us all. Its conquest deserves the best of all mankind, and its opportunity for peaceful cooperation may never come again. But why, some say, elevate health above politics and culture? Why choose this as our goal? And they may well ask Why climb the highest mountain? Why, 62 years ago, fly to the moon? Why does Vanderbilt play Tennessee in football?

We choose to fix health. We choose to start by Ending Heart Disease in this decade and do the other things, not because they are easy, but because they are hard, because that goal will serve to organize and measure the best of our energies and skills, because this challenge is one that we are willing to accept, one we are unwilling to postpone, and one which we intend to win.

It is for these reasons that I regard the decision today to shift our efforts in health from low to high gear as among the most important decisions that will be made in our lives.

Definition of Ending Heart Disease by 2035:

Heart disease is the #1 cause of death for men, women, and people of most racial and ethnic groups, according to the CDC. One person dies every 34 seconds from cardiovascular disease, and about 33% of all mortality in the US is caused by heart disease. The disease is also expensive, costing over $400 billion per year. To hold ourselves accountable, we must clearly define what we mean by "End Heart Disease."

To significantly reduce the prevalence and impact of heart disease in the US by 2035, with a measurable target of removing it from the top five causes of death as listed in the US government statistics of all-cause mortality. For reference, heart disease has been the #1 cause of death since we have been tracking causes of mortality.

> <u>One Clear Metric:</u>
> The rank of heart disease as a cause of death in the US - currently #1. We will celebrate the "End of Heart Disease" when it has fallen out of the top 5 causes of death.

Scouting the Enemy: Understanding Heart Disease

To be successful in stopping it or finding a cure, we must work to understand this disease fully. Heart disease is the leading cause of death worldwide, a stark reality underscored by the fact that someone dies from cardiovascular disease roughly every 34 seconds in the United States. But what exactly is heart disease, and why does it affect so many? Cardiovascular disease (aka heart disease) encompasses a range of conditions affecting the heart and blood vessels, from coronary artery disease to heart failure. As a first step in our journey to end heart disease, we explore its causes and, most importantly, develop ways to reduce symptoms and eventually stop it from killing so many of our friends, family, and Elevate Health 2050 Members.

At the center of many cardiovascular issues lies atherosclerosis, a process where plaque builds up inside the arteries. This plaque, composed of cholesterol and other components, narrows the arteries, reducing blood flow. A helpful analogy is a water pipe. The water flows along the inside of the pipe. If something, such as soap, grease, or food waste, builds up along the inside of the pipe over many years, then water cannot flow as quickly and easily within the pipe. At first, the debris will not cause much of a problem. The water will meet the obstacle but easily flow around it. Over time, as more of the pipe becomes blocked, water will flow more slowly along the pipe, and eventually it will become completely clogged. This is in effect the same process that occurs in our cardiovascular system. Atherosclerosis is the medical term for the "building up of plaque" along the vessels that carry blood throughout the body.

This gradual process of plaque accumulation typically begins in childhood and progresses over 30-40 years. Often, the patient has no symptoms, which is one of the most challenging issues in the treatment of heart disease. Atherosclerosis usually can be first seen in teenagers or even young children as fatty streaks in the aorta, which is the largest artery in the body. This early damage is asymptomatic, so typically the patient is unaware.

Natural Human Repairs with Calcium

As we age into our 20s and 30s, the plaque buildup continues, but there are still no clear symptoms for most patients. The streaks become thicker with the accumulation of cholesterol and other fatty substances. The body has a process to repair the inside of the blood vessels. It builds a structure to cover up and control the damage by creating fibrous calcified plaques. This "repair job" stabilizes the blood vessels and repairs the immediate damage. However, the fiber and hard calcium also stiffen the vessel, making it less flexible to expand and move with the body. This makes the entire cardiovascular system slightly more fragile, not in the sense that it will break, but less resilient and able to adjust to physical exertion or other factors that apply stress to the system. In addition, these repairs add to the size of the plaque on the inside of the vessel. This accelerates the negative impact on the patient's blood flow.

Since these fibrous calcified plaques are the only reason calcium is found in the vessels, we can use the calcium screen to determine how many of these repairs the patient's body has been forced to use to repair the blood vessels. If a patient has a calcium score of 0, this means they have no evidence of atherosclerotic repair. However, when we find calcium present in the vessels, we know the body has been repairing damage. Since there are no early symptoms of heart disease, the calcium score is an inexpensive and convenient way to screen for heart disease.

When these narrowed arteries supply the heart muscle itself, it leads to coronary artery disease. This means the arteries supplying blood flow, oxygen, and other nutrients to the heart itself lose efficacy, causing stress and eventually problems for the heart. Blockages in these arteries can cause angina. Angina is the medical term for chest pain due to reduced blood flow to the heart itself. It can feel like a squeezing, pressure, heaviness, tightness, or pain in the chest. If the narrowing of the artery continues, it may become totally blocked. If a complete blockage occurs, it cuts off the oxygen to the heart, resulting in damage to the heart muscle tissue. This is a heart attack, or in medical terminology, a myocardial infarction.

Other Less-Common Types of Heart Disease

In addition to atherosclerosis, there are two other ways the heart can develop an issue and fail to pump enough blood to meet the body's needs. This is called Heart Failure, and it has two primary causes: arrhythmias and structural issues.

Arrhythmias are defined as irregular heart rhythms. In this case, the heart is structurally sound, but it fails to "beat properly." A healthy heart contracts and relaxes in a consistent, beating rhythm. It is this contraction and relaxation in the proper rhythm that pumps the blood out of one chamber and into the next, and then out to the body. Arrhythmias describe the state of improper rhythm such that either the heart is "out of sync," essentially beating out of rhythm or the heart fails to execute a full contract and release cycle.

Structural heart disease is defined as a heart that has grown into the wrong shape or has a part that is not working properly. It can be the case that one of the heart chambers has grown too large and extended to allow for effective pumping. Alternatively, patients can develop problems with the heart valves. These valves are one-way openings between the different chambers of the heart. Valves must open at the proper time to allow blood to flow out to the next chamber, and then they must close to allow the chamber to refill properly. If a valve becomes damaged, the heart can lose its ability to move blood, negatively impacting function.

Changing Our Perspective

In his book Outlive, Peter Attia argues that relying on a "10-year risk" assessment for chronic diseases is a dangerously short-sighted approach. He believes this standard medical practice, which only predicts your risk for things like heart attack or stroke over the next decade, misses the long-term, insidious nature of chronic illness. This 10-year window of time is too short for diseases that begin decades earlier and worsen over time, such as heart disease. Instead, he advocates for a proactive, long-term strategy he calls Medicine 3.0. We agree and plan to proactively apply these ideas to heart disease specifically.

We take the perspective that our goal is to end heart disease altogether. From this point of view, ten years of safety is insufficient. Instead, we want to measure each Member's risk of death by heart disease as opposed to another cause of death. There is no time horizon, except to say that heart disease is currently the number 1-ranked cause of death across every member type. One of the first scientific questions we aim to address is how to measure and map the actual risk of cardiovascular death for each member, thereby attracting people to join our cause and help. We want to lower the risk.

The current Medicine 2.0 approach to heart disease is too passive and slow. In the US, physicians are taught to use a 10-year risk score for cardiovascular disease (CVD). Although this tool has improved since its development in 1998, it requires an update. This risk score is rooted in the long-running Framingham Heart Study and includes key factors like age, sex, total and HDL cholesterol, blood pressure, smoking status, and diabetes. The risk score was updated and revised in 2008 to predict a broader range of cardiovascular events, including stroke and heart failure, in addition to CVD. We assert that 10 years is not a long enough timeline for most patients. If you are 40 years old, it is not very important to determine your risk of having a heart attack, stroke, or death due to coronary heart disease before age 50. Rather, it is more valuable to understand your risk over the next 40 years - before age 80. This would be the patient's actual risk of death by heart disease.

Prioritize Early Screening

The core idea of the End Heart Disease initiative is that heart disease primarily kills people through 20-30 years of accumulation of relatively minor negative changes to the patient's overall cardiovascular system. The hardest part of treating Heart Disease is that this damage causes no negative symptoms for the patient. Typically, they are not aware that anything is wrong until the disease has progressed to a dangerous level. Certainly, there are exceptions, but we believe we reduce CVD deaths by over 50% through early screening and treatment. While this will not be enough to knock heart disease out of the top 5 causes of mortality, it will save millions of lives and give early momentum to the End Heart Disease by 2035 initiative.

Identifying patients with early signs of Heart Disease will allow us to get them into proper care and halt this accumulation of damage. End Heart Disease will launch a widely publicized campaign offering a free coronary artery calcium (CAC) screening test for anyone 35 years of age or older. The campaign's messaging will emphasize the test's ability to provide a definitive, “black-and-white” result. The CAC score test is a 20-minute, non-invasive CT scan of the heart. It measures the amount of calcium in the coronary arteries, which is a direct measure of atherosclerosis (calcified plaque buildup). These calcified plaques are the body's natural method to repair damage to blood vessels. If a patient has a positive CAC score, it means their body has already been repairing damage related to Heart Disease. A score of zero means no calcified plaque is present, while a positive score indicates the presence of plaque.

A CAC test is relatively affordable, with costs ranging from $75 to $150 per patient, depending on the provider and location. It is not typically covered by insurance, but we plan to make it the primary diagnostic screen. For the purposes of this chapter, we will use an average cost of $100 per CAC test for our calculations.

Illustrating the Power of Elevate Health Markets

While the CAC screening is relatively inexpensive, we can use this project to illustrate the power of the Elevate Health Community and market design. In 1990, there were slightly over 4.1 million babies born in the US. This is important because these people are now 35 years old. Of course, not all of these people will learn of the End Heart Disease project, and others may learn of it but not engage. Still, older people will also sign up to be screened. To keep things as simple as possible, we assume that we can screen 5% of 35-year-olds; this gives us a rough estimate of 205,000 people to screen in 2026. At $100 per person, this will cost $20.5 million in CAC screening expenses in he first year.. How can we afford this investment? Luckily, the Elevate Health market is set up to navigate this type of investment in the overall health of the community.

Returning to Our Personas

As we described in Chapter 5, our four personas: Heather, Andy, Paul, and Ellie, join the Elevate Health Community to get a free "Heart Health Calcium Screen." The process works as follows: any interested person aged 35 or older simply completes a 3-question intake form, providing their name, phone number, and date of birth. Then they book an appointment for the screening.

Within 24 hours after the screening, they are welcomed to the Elevate Health Community via text message by their new Personal Wellness AI-Coach. The onboarding is designed to be easy and fun. The AI-Coach's role is to learn about the member and assist them in clarifying and then working toward their goals. Using the calcium score, Elevate Health places each Member on one of two paths. If the Calcium Score is 0, the AI-Coach knows the Member is low risk for heart disease. It gives them this great news and asks if they have any other health and wellness goals. However, if the Calcium Score is positive, the Wellness Coach knows the member has some existing heart disease. It uses the exact CA score to estimate the severity of the disease and helps the member understand that heart disease typically develops slowly over many decades. The bad news is that the Member has some evidence of Heart Disease, but the good news is that by catching it early, they have several effective treatment options. Once the AI-Coach educates the member and takes some additional key data points, such as "do they smoke?", "what is their height & weight?", and "have they ever had a cholesterol test?" The member has the option to find an appropriate physician independently or use one of the options available in the Elevate Health 2050 Community.

Members with Heart Disease Referred to Cargivers

Heart disease patients are some of the most valuable patients to a health system, and they will drive gross margins well over the 15% level, putting these organizations in the Elevate Health High-margin category. Of course, each Member will receive individualized care to meet their specific situation, but we can make some basic assumptions. Reimbursable services with most insurance plans will be slightly higher for commercial plans than CMS pays for Medicare patients. However, it is easier to find published rates for Medicare, so we use these rates, which may be slightly conservative.

The first visit to the cardiologist is a comprehensive evaluation. This involves a detailed history, physical exam, and discussion of the CAC score and next steps. CMS reimbursement for a new patient office visit can range from $200 to $400, depending on the complexity of the medical decision-making. We will select the midpoint of $300. For reference, we are using the CMS CPT codes, including 99204-99215. The physician will also order a comprehensive set of blood tests, including a full lipid panel, A1C, and other inflammatory markers. The reimbursement for these labs is typically a few dollars per test, totaling $100 to $200. We will select the midpoint of $150. Often, the cardiologist will likely order further tests to understand the functional impact of the plaque. This could involve an Echocardiogram, which is a non-invasive ultrasound of the heart that assesses its structure and function. CMS reimbursement is typically in the range of ~$400 (CPT code 93306).

Depending on the progression of the disease, the physician may also order a Stress Test (CPT code 93015). This test evaluates the heart's function under stress. The reimbursement for a full stress test, including the physician supervision and interpretation, is approximately $350. For our purposes, we will assume the doctor skips this test.

However, the physician will benefit from the long-term revenue stream related to managing this member over time. Most doctors will prescribe medications such as a statin to lower cholesterol and possibly a blood pressure medication. While the pharmacy gets the medication revenue, the physician's role is in the ongoing management and prescription renewals. Follow-up office visits (CPT codes 99213-99214) are typically reimbursed in the $100-$250 range. A typical patient might have 2-4 of these visits per year. We assume one additional patient visit to the clinic at $150. It may be necessary to perform some extra procedures, depending on the CAC score as well as the other test results. The patient may require more intensive procedures. For example, a CT Angiogram is a more advanced diagnostic imaging technique to visualize the coronary arteries. CMS reimbursement is approximately $400 (CPT code 75574). We assume this is not required.

Estimated First-Year Reimbursement

Clinic visit: $300

Lab tabs:$150

Echocardiogram: $400

Stress test: NA

Follow-up clinic visit: $150

Total: $1,000

10% Community reinvestment: $100

This allows us to earn $100 toward the cost of the next CAC screen. However, this figure is just for the first year and assumes no significant events. As you can see, the reimbursement for a single patient can generate a consistent and significant revenue stream for a health system over time. However, the actual value of heart disease patients lies in the long-term value. A managed heart disease patient is a predictable source of revenue through routine visits and occasional diagnostic tests, avoiding the massive, but unpredictable, costs associated with a heart attack. If the Member were to have a heart attack, it would increase the revenue to the physician; however, we want to avoid this outcome, so we do not plan for it.

This is a strong initial step, but we only expect 50% of our new Members to have heart disease, yet 100% of them will incur the $100 CAC screening cost. Thus, we need to find about $200 for each heart disease patient in order to recoup the screening expense of three new members fully. To reach this goal, we return to the RPM aspects of Fueling the Elevate Flywheel.

Remote Patient Monitoring Utility

As the Member interacts with the AI-Coach, learns about their heart disease, and begins a relationship with a qualified physician, the AI seamlessly guides them through the process of fulfilling Remote Patient Monitoring (RPM) requirements, either by CMS if they are over 65 or commercial insurance if they are younger. Medicare reimburses Elevate Health's Foundations a monthly fee of approximately $120 to monitor the health and wellness of Members with heart disease.

As a Low-Margin service, Foundations keep gross margins below 15%. Therefore, our Member will receive benefits on average worth $102/month. This can take the form of assembling their healthcare digital twin, participating in exercise classes, or joining a healthy eating class. Since the Personal AI-Coach already manages the Member's health identity, data, and rights, the cost to the Member is negligible. Therefore, the increase in Member Surplus related to the RPM Service is about $100/month. However, the remaining $18/month can be used to offset the initial CAC screening costs. Therefore, the full $200 will be paid off after 6 months. In this way, our End Heart Disease project will be able to generate enough cash flow to continue to offer free calcium screening to all new members in a sustainable manner.

Early Screening and Physician Care - not enough

While the push to screen and treat 100% of people over the age of 35 will have a dramatically positive impact on cardiac care and reduce deaths related to heart disease, we do not expect it to be fast enough to hit our 2035 goal. Even if we can screen and treat 100% of 35-year-olds AND we make the assumption that once under long-term physician care, none of these patients will die of heart disease, it won't be enough. Most heart attacks and related deaths occur after the age of 50, so in ten years, none of our screened 35-year-olds will be that old. This strategy will build awareness and save lives, but it will not be sufficient to End Heart Disease by 2035.

To achieve our goal of ending heart disease within 10 years, we will need to find creative new approaches and treatments to combat the disease.   This was true for the Moon Mission in 1962, and it is true for our "moonshot project." However, we have five categories of where we expect to leverage the coming 3 waves of innovation to help beat heart disease for good.

Research & Innovation:

We also plan to use our End Heart Disease project as a means to focus the Elevate Health Community on research projects related to the effective treatment of all types of Heart Disease. One of the options for High-Margin Organizations to reinvest back into our community will be to designate some or all of these funds to the End Heart Disease Project.

Tokenized Research Funding:

These funds will be used to create an Endowment to benefit the End Heart Disease Heart Tokens. Each year, we will invest this Endowment in USD and BTC and use the proceeds (5%) to send out Cash to fund research projects in the form of 1Heart= $1. These Heart tokens can be used as equal to $1 on the Elevate Health Settlement payment processing utility. Members and Foundations that share our passion to End Heart Disease are encouraged to invest in the End Heart Disease Project alongside the Elevate Health Community. Our hope is that as we gain awareness in the US market for our Calcium Screening 35 year 35-year-olds, we will attract others to join in our moonshot vision.

Open-Source Collaboration:

Encourage data sharing and collaboration among researchers through decentralized platforms, accelerating progress. We may also experiment with offering Heart Tokens to Members willing to share their personal health data as long as it is never segmented into groups smaller than 100 Members. Since we know the Members will have to respend the Hearts back into the community of Caregivers, we may find this to be an effective way to gather a large amount of data while engaging many diverse members of our community.

Badges as NFTs:

Over time, we plan to develop unique badges to recognize significant contributions, milestones achieved, and project successes. These badges are NFTs and held in the members' identities. They also may convey rights to community benefits or unique experiences.

Impact Reports:

Provide regular, transparent reports on project progress and the movement of impact metrics, demonstrating the tangible results of all the efforts across the End Heart Disease by 2035 Project.

Summary

All moonshot projects look impossible at the start. When Kennedy predicted that "the US would land a man on the moon before the end of this decade," no one knew if or how the US could achieve this seemingly impossible goal. Yet the vision captivated our country during Neil Howes's last High Period. You know the end of the story. Science, math, and engineering students set to work and invented rockets, plastics, and the internet.

Heart Disease is the biggest killer of all diseases. We do not know how to end the disease in 10 years. We believe our early screening and proactive treatment will stop all future 35-year-olds from dying of heart disease. This will end the disease but not for 50 years or so - when today's 35-year-olds are 85. At that point, there will be no untreated heart disease. However, to succeed in 10 years, now that is much more engaging. First of all, it may help me personally, and definitely my kids and grandkids will benefit. Sendond, we now need to dream, create, and invent. This is America's best trait. Unfortunately, we need to be called to adventure in order us to find the creative spark.

Return to Table of Contents

www.ingramcontent.com/pod-product-compliance
Lightning Source LLC
LaVergne TN
LVHW052030200926
848481LV00005B/1636